UNIVERS ... EPEN
... AM
WIT... N
FROM THE LIBRARY

D0272108

DATE D'

AN ESSAY

MEDICAL, PHILOSOPHICAL, AND CHEMICAL

ON DRUNKENNESS

AND ITS EFFECTS ON THE HUMAN BODY

Tavistock Classics
in the History of Psychiatry

GENERAL EDITORS:

W.F. Bynum and Roy Porter

Current interest in the history of psychiatry is growing rapidly both among the psychiatric profession and social historians. This new series is designed to bring back into print many classic documents from earlier centuries. Each reprint has been chosen for the series because of its social and intellectual significance, and includes a substantial introduction written by an eminent scholar in the history of psychiatry.

Lifes Preservative Against Self-Killing (1637)
by John Sym (*ed.* Michael MacDonald)

Illustrations of Madness (1810)
by John Haslam (*ed.* Roy Porter)

Observations on Maniacal Disorders (1792)
by William Pargeter (*ed.* Stanley W. Jackson)

AN ESSAY

MEDICAL, PHILOSOPHICAL, AND CHEMICAL

ON DRUNKENNESS

AND ITS EFFECTS ON THE HUMAN BODY

BY

THOMAS TROTTER

Edited with an Introduction by

Roy Porter

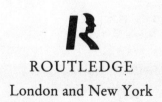

ROUTLEDGE

London and New York

MEDICAL LIBRARY
QUEEN'S MEDICAL CENTRE

Class	WM 10 TRO
Fund	ZJA 911
Book No.	6200446670

√c

First published 1988
by Routledge
11 New Fetter Lane, London EC4P 4EE
29 West 35th Street, New York, NY 10001

© 1988 Introduction by Roy Porter

Printed in Great Britain at the University Press, Cambridge

All rights reserved. No part of this book may be reprinted or reproduced or utilized
in any form or by any electronic, mechanical, or other means, now known or
hereafter invented, including photocopying and recording, or in any information
storage or retrieval system, without permission in writing from the publishers.

British Library Cataloguing in Publication Data

Trotter, Thomas
    An essay, medical, philosophical, and
    chemical on drunkenness and its effects on
    the human body.
    1. Man. Physiology. Effects of alcohol
    I. Title II. Series
    615'.7828

Library of Congress Cataloging in Publication Data

Trotter, Thomas, 1760–1832.
    An essay, medical, philosophical, and chemical, on drunkenness and
its effects on the human body / Thomas Trotter; editor with an
introduction by Roy Porter.
        p.   cm.—(Tavistock classics in the history of psychiatry)
    Reprint. Orginally published: London: Printed for Longman,
Hurst, Rees, and Orme, 1804.
    Includes index.
    ISBN 0–415–00636–8
    1. Alcoholism—Early works to 1800.   2. Alcohol—Physiological
effect—Early works to 1800.   I. Porter, Roy, 1946– . II. Title.
III. Series.
    [DNLM: WM T858e 1804a]
RC565.T76 1988
616.86'1—dc 19
DNLM/DLC
for Library of Congress

ISBN 0–415–00636–8

CONTENTS

PREFACE

The Tavistock Classics in the History of Psychiatry series meets a considerable need amongst academics, practitioners, and all those who are more broadly interested in the development of psychiatry. Psychiatry as a discipline has always paid considerable heed to its own founders, its history, and emergent traditions. It is one field in which the relevance of the past to the present does not diminish. There is a high professional awareness of the history of the subject, and many aspects of this are now benefiting from fruitful dialogue with the now rapidly expanding investigations of historians and historical sociologists.

Yet two factors greatly hamper our grasp of psychiatry's past. On the one hand, a considerable number of the formative texts on the rise of psychiatry are exceedingly difficult to obtain, even from libraries. As a small discipline in earlier centuries, many of the major works were published only in short runs, and many, even of the classics, have never been reprinted at all. This present series aims to overcome this problem, by making available a selection of such key works. Mostly they are books originally published in the English language; in other cases where the original language was, say, French or German, we are reprinting contemporary English translations; in a few cases, we hope to present entirely new translations of classic Continental works.

On the other hand, in many instances little is commonly known of the life and ideas of the authors of these texts, and their works have never been subjected to thorough analyses. Our intention in this series is to follow the model of the now defunct Dawson series of psychiatric reprints, edited and introduced by Richard Hunter

and Ida Macalpine, now, alas, both dead, and to provide substantial
scholarly introductions to each volume, based upon original research.
Thus the book and its author will illuminate each other, and one
will avoid the dilemma of a text isolated in an intellectual vacuum,
or simply the accumulation of miscellaneous biographical data. It is
our hope that this series will break new ground in the history of
psychiatry, and secure a new readership for a number of illustrative
works in psychiatry's rich and fascinating past.

INTRODUCTION

Roy Porter

Through much of Europe and North America it was the first half of the nineteenth century which saw the dawn of modern society. Population mushroomed at a hitherto unknown rate, leading to the emergence of gigantic new conurbations. The demands of commercial and industrial capitalism brought into being in these manufacturing towns, mining areas and ports a concentrated proletarianised work force, typically uprooted from traditional social ties and patterns. And alongside the metaphorical armies of navvies who built the canals and railways were the real armies and navies which fought the Napoleonic Wars and later served the military designs of the new nation states.

Mass society was thus born; and one of its features – indeed, one of its terrifying problems, as contemporaries never ceased to point out – was mass drunkenness. There was, of course, nothing new in the heavy consumption of alcoholic beverages, nothing new in drunkenness, as the lives of people real and fictional from Noah through Falstaff to James Boswell make abundantly clear.[1] In traditional rural society it was good housekeeping to brew or distil grain surpluses into ale or spirits; and given the impure nature of the water supply, fermented beverages formed safe as well as warming, nourishing and convivial drinks. Ale houses and inns were the foci of community life ('a tavern chair', reflected Samuel Johnson, 'is the throne of human felicity'). The well-off marked their good fortune with the conspicuous hospitality of the free-flowing bowl, while the poor forgot their troubles, their lives of incessant grinding toil and poverty, in the Bacchanalian culture of carnival, when, on May Day, at Harvest Home, or at Christmas and New Year, peasants were permitted to booze themselves into oblivion.[2]

Introduction by Roy Porter

Pre-industrial Europe abounded with warnings, religious, moral and medical, about the dangers of the demon drink: in tippling, as in everything else, moderation was the golden rule. But root-and-branch hostility to alcoholic liquor as such – as distinct from its abuses and excesses – was highly exceptional; there were few Malvolios, urging total prohibition in cakes and ale. After all, through the Eucharist, the taking of wine was validated within the ceremonial and sacramental rituals of the Christian churches (contrast the fierce prohibitions of Islam), and as the great American puritan, Increase Mather, had put it, 'drink is in itself a good creature of God'. Similarly, traditional medical opinion, both learned and folk, regarded wine as a valuable cordial, a view spelt out at length in Dr Peter Shaw's *The Juice of the Grape, or Wine Preferable to Water* (1724). Many of the tried-and-tested items of the pharmacopoeia were alcohol-based, as also were the patent and proprietary nostrums which began to flood the medical self-care market during the eighteenth century.[3]

Down the centuries critics, of course, tiraded against tippling; but drunkenness was typically treated as a problem which was individual, local, and temporary, confined to times of feast and festivities, rather than a real threat to social survival itself. The solutions were thought to lie in personal discipline and in specific measures of social control (the suppression of a rowdy fair, the closing of notorious drinking-dens and so forth).[4]

Events, however, took a far more ominous turn during the eighteenth century. In certain regions of Europe, advances in capitalist agriculture were by then producing occasional huge grain supplies. The upshot was that great towns became flooded with really cheap spirits; during the 'gin craze' in London between the 1730s and the 1750s there were at one point 8,000 dram shops in the capital, and one could notoriously get drunk for a penny and dead drunk for twopence. Labourers who could never have afforded to get blotto on ale descended into constant stupefaction – and beyond, into the grave – on cheap gin. Some thirteen million gallons of gin were consumed in 1734; by 1742 the total was nineteen million. The demoralizing, indeed fatal, effects were all too visible on the streets. In its most acute aspects, the gin craze proved only temporary. Governments acted to raise duties and curb the gin-shops, while a steadily rising population quickly put an end to the grain mountain.[5]

Nevertheless the gin craze – most famously depicted of course in Hogarth's print, 'Gin Lane' – did mark the shape of things to come, registering the moment at which ardent spirits became the real menace, and brewing and distilling emerged as big businesses within market capitalism. Traditionally the rich had kept their cellars full of wine and the lower orders guzzled their home- or village-brewed beer. During the eighteenth century, however, stronger liquors came into vogue. Port was brought in cheaply from Portugal, brandy was smuggled from France; gin was adopted from Holland in the late seventeenth century; with the rise of the sugar plantations, rum ('grog') became a favourite drink of sailors and colonials, and home-distilled whisky swept North America. Potent, dangerous, and often extremely cheap, the spread of ardent spirits raised the problem of drunkenness onto a new plane.

Danger also lurked in the contemporaneous emergence of the great capitalist brewers – entrepreneurs such as Henry Thrale or Samuel Whitbread, who operated on a scale comparable to the greatest factory-owning cotton-spinner or mines magnate. Commercial brewers naturally wished to mass produce. This meant developing types of ales which would travel well and have a long storage life. The creation of the heavy 'porters' answered this need. But 'porter' was certainly more intoxicating than the traditional lighter ales, and critics – Thomas Trotter was one of them – commonly alleged that such brewers adulterated their products with noxious additives used both as stabilizing agents and perhaps to create addiction. Thus by the close of the eighteenth century, the alcoholic drinks available were more potent and perilous than previously.[6]

These developments of course paved the way for the massive surge of heavy drinking which ultra-rapid urban and industrial growth, with its ready money and social disruption, inevitably created in the nineteenth century. The new drink problem was a phenomenon tabulated by social statisticians, deplored by moralists and preachers, and analysed by commentators, who associated the evils of the bottle with every mode of vice and crime, above all with prostitution, violence and (mainly later in the century) physical and psychic degeneracy. Charitable organizations – the remote fore-runners of Alcoholics Anonymous – sprang up to warn about the demon drink, to save the sot, and to provide alternative forms of recreation. For the first time, organized temperance movements were launched, aiming to win converts to the cause of complete abstinence, and, especially in the USA, to prohibition. And, not least, the massive new prominence of drunkenness, with all its attendant disorders, diseases and accidents, attracted the public alarm of the medical profession for the first time.[7]

Building to some degree on the work of precursors such as Erasmus Darwin, nineteenth century doctors set about investigating the pathology of excessive drinking, exploring its associations with conditions such as dropsy, heart disease, cirrhosis of the liver (newly described by Dr Matthew Baillie), nervous disorders, paralyses and, of course, sudden and premature death. Habitual drunkenness was shown to be critical in the aetiology of particular diseases, such as apoplexy; and the emergent psychiatric profession underlined the causal links between chronic drunkenness and insanity (the vast Victorian expansion of lunatic asylums, which readily filled up with inebriates, made such relationships crystal clear).[8] From the early nineteenth century, particular syndromes were newly labelled, ascribable to alcohol abuse, notably *delirium tremens*, first described by Thomas Sutton in 1813, and more fully discussed by Samuel Burton Pearson under the name of 'brain fever'.[9]

Thus doctors explored how heavy drinking caused disorder and disease. More challenging was the claim advanced frequently in the first half of the nineteenth century that heavy and persistent alcohol consumption was itself a disease in its own right, or at least a key symptom of some underlying disease. In other words, just as one would speak of a consumptive or an epileptic as someone suffering from a serious ailment, so the habitual drunkard was equally to be regarded as a diseased person, falling within the province of medicine to diagnose and treat. Thus the drunkard – a wretch traditionally seen as suffering from moral or religious weakness – came to be medicalized, and the 'disease concept' of drunkenness was crystalized, leading by the mid-nineteenth century to the notion of the disease of 'alcoholism' and of the 'alcoholic' as a suitable case for medical attention.[10]

It is important not to oversimplify the formulation of the disease concept of alcoholism. There was not one single concept but many, and the various approaches all had their insights and merits. One viewpoint was advanced by the German physician, C. von Brühl-

Cramer (d. 1821), who argued in his influential *Über die Trunksucht und eine rationelle Heilmethode derselben* that the propensity to excessive drinking was a symptom of a physical disease (*Trunksucht*, or dipsomania). Thus drinking to excess should be seen not as a vice, but rather as analogous to the power of fevers to create unslakable thirsts; Brühl-Cramer also suggested parallels with pica, the inordinate longings of pregnant women for peculiar food or drink. Regarding what he called 'dipsomania' as a physical disease of the whole nervous system, Brühl-Cramer recommended treatment with physical medicines.[11]

A different viewpoint lay in treating excessive drinking essentially as a *mental* disease, or more frequently perhaps as the *symptom* of mental disorder. The leading French psychiatrist, J. E. D. Esquirol (1772–1840), thus assimilated habitual drunkenness into his favoured category of monomania. Just as some people, sane in other respects, had deluded perceptions and ungovernable appetites with regard to property, power or sex, so others were possessed by irresistible impulses to drink. Esquirol noted the close affinities between drunkenness and insanity; but unlike most asylum keepers he was less concerned to blame drink as the cause of madness than to point out how habitual drinking was a tell-tale sign of underlying mental disturbance. Esquirol's interpretation has some similarities to that developed in the 1830s by the German physician, Karl Rosch (1808–66), who regarded habitual drunkenness as typically the outcome of the combination of psychological predisposition (inner temperament) with social circumstances (squalid housing, bad company, etc).[12]

Yet another approach was adopted by perhaps the most eminent investigator of drunkenness, the Swede, Magnus Huss (1807–90), who was responsible for coining the term 'alcoholism' in 1852. Huss approached the problem primarily as a clinician. He investigated sensory, motor and psychic disturbances, and offered a particularly acute account of the neurological symptoms of the chronic alcoholic: nausea, convulsions, ringing of the ears, vertigo, and so forth. Huss was sceptical about identifying underlying psychological causes of alcohol habituation, and specifically denied the view, then being developed by 'degenerationist' psychiatrists such as Morel, that the alcoholic diathesis was in itself heritable.[13]

Thomas Trotter and the History of Alcoholism

The first half of the nineteenth century thus saw chronic drunkenness – eventually 'alcoholism' – firmly established upon the map as a medical disorder. Thomas Trotter's traditional claim to historical fame is that he was the first to outline – albeit not finally to formulate – many of the viewpoints and strategies subsequently adumbrated in the writings of Brühl-Cramer, Rosch, Esquirol, Huss and others. Brian Harrison, historian of the Victorian temperance movement, has thus written, 'Trotter was the first scientific investigator of drunkenness';[14] and it is significant that he has been credited with the ultimate accolade of a Garrison and Morton number (currently 2071.1), identifying him as the Columbus of the medical study of drunkenness. There is no doubt that Trotter's work made a splash; his major treatise, the *Essay, Medical, Philosophical, and Chemical, on Drunkenness*, published in 1804, went through further editions in 1807, 1810 and 1812; it saw an American version in 1813, and was also translated into German and Swedish.

There is much truth in the traditional view that the *Essay ... on Drunkenness* was a notable, original and pioneering work. Trotter quite explicitly, indeed aggressively, defines drunkenness as a medical prerogative, noting condescendingly that parsons and moralists have long had their crack at the drink problem, but it must properly be the labour of the medical profession to solve it.[15] He categorically states that excessive drinking is a 'disease';[16] indeed quite specifically a mental disease.[17] A substantial part of his treatise is devoted to accounts of the symptoms and sequelae of the syndrome; but Trotter was no narrow clinician, and he showed himself acutely attentive to the sociopsychological circumstances which favoured heavy drinking. His 200-page book effectively sketchmapped the field.

Thus Trotter deserves attention as a major forerunner of nineteenth-century students of alcoholism. But he believed he had a grander claim to fame. For he regarded himself as the very first doctor to collar the problem of habitual drunkenness. He informs us at the commencement of his book that when he was choosing the topic for his Edinburgh University MD dissertation, he was anxious to ensure that he would pick one which had 'never been noticed by any former graduate' – one, indeed, 'only cursorily' dealt with in the medical literature at large; and at numerous points in his text he trumpets his own originality: 'I have not any precursors in my labours'.[18]

There is some warrant for Trotter's belief in his own novelty. Drunkenness had, of course, figured large in writings ever since Antiquity, and there was a sizeable body of sermons, advice books, works of self-improvement and so forth, in English, on the subject. Various medical practitioners in Enlightenment England had written papers dealing with drunkenness, or had discussed drinking as part of the wider questions of regimen and diet, matters contained within the traditional framework of the 'non-naturals'. Bernard Mandeville, George Cheyne and John Coakley Lettsom are amongst the most eminent who examined the pathology of hard drinking, but the subject of alcohol abuse was at least touched upon by scores of medical writers, as for instance William Buchan in his much-read *Domestic Medicine*.[19] Mad-doctors blamed drunkenness in their aetiologies of insanity, and, not surprisingly, many practitioners commented upon the evils of the 'gin craze'. Even so, Trotter's treatise seems to have been the first book-length analysis of drunkenness by a British doctor – though it should not be forgotten that the American, Benjamin Rush's influential *An Inquiry into the Effects of Ardent Spirits Upon the Human Body* (1785), had already appeared, a work to which Trotter curiously seems never to refer.[20]

Trotter presents a forthrightly medical view of the condition: 'I consider Drunkenness, strictly speaking, to be a disease', an idea he later refines into the province of psychiatry ('the habit of drunkenness is a disease of the mind').[21] The striking clarity of this formulation is probably original. But it does not seem as if the ideas underlying it were really breaking new ground. For it was not uncommon for British practitioners earlier in the eighteenth century to construe drunkenness as a medical problem (rather than simply as a moral, religious or legal weakness), and the term 'disease' and its cognates had already been deployed in this context by physicians such as George Cheyne and Anthony Fothergill. Moreover, Trotter's perceptive grasp of the psychological underpinnings of habitual drunkenness – showing how the mind becomes enslaved to its own desires – was hardly so original as he thought. Very similar notions of the formation of chains of habits had already been outlined by his predecessors. Some twenty years before Trotter, John Coakley Lettsom had offered a comparable vision of the fatal downward spiral, leading from tippling for stimulus, relief or exhilaration, to low spirits, which were its inevitable after effects; which in turn could be obliterated only by further bouts of yet heavier drinking. Lettsom gave as an example[22]

> those of delicate habits, who have endeavoured to overcome their nervous debility by the aid of spirits: many of these have begun the use of these poisons from persuasions of their utility, rather than from love of them: the relief, however, being temporary, to keep up their effects, frequent access is had to the same delusion, till at length what was taken by compulsion, gains attachment, and a little drop of brandy, or gin and water, becomes as necessary as food; the female sex, from natural delicacy, acquire this custom by small degrees, and the poison being admitted in small doses, is slow in its operations, but not less painful in its effects.

Eventually, Lettsom argued, such dependence would set in that

> neither threats nor persuasions are powerful enough to overcome it, and the miserable sufferer is so infatuated, as in spite of locks and keys, to bribe by high rewards the dependent nurse, privately to procure the fatal draught.

Moreover, some fifty years before Lettsom, George Cheyne had been advancing comparable ideas, showing how old soaks eventually succumbed to alcohol 'cravings':[23]

> They begin with the weaker wines; These, by Use and Habit, will not do; They leave the Stomach sick and mawkish; they fly to stronger Wines, and stronger still, and run the Climax from Brandy to Barbados Waters, and double-distill'd Spirits, till at last they find nothing hot enough for them.

Thus, as Cheyne saw it, the slavery of 'Necessity upon Necessity' set in, moving from 'Drops to Drams', through which in time 'Drams beget more Drams ... so that at last the miserable Creature suffers a true Martyrdom'.[24]

And before Cheyne, Bernard Mandeville had offered a graphic account of the demon drink and the slide into alcohol addiction, putting his version of the 'Sot's Progress' into the mouth of a fictional character, 'Misomedon', who recounted how the drinker made rods for his own back. 'Misomedon' first praised the bottle god:[25]

> It has laid my pains, appeas'd my Soul, made me forget my Sorrows, and fancy over night, that all my afflictions had left me; but the next Morning, before the Strength of the Charm has been quite worn off, they have in Crowds return'd upon me with a Vengeance and my self paid dearly for the deceitful Cure. 'Tis unspeakable in what Confusion and Horror, Guilt, Fear, and Repentance I have wak'd, in what depth of Grief, Fear, Anguish and Misery my Spirits have been sunk, or how forlorn and destitute of all Hopes and Comforts I have sometimes thought my self after the Use of this fallacious remedy.

It would be easy to multiply instances, from British and Continental physicians alike, of an awareness of the interplay between psyche, habit and alcohol dependence before the appearance of Trotter's work, for such perceptions were not unique to doctors but were part of common experience. For instance, Samuel Johnson – at one stage a heavy drinker – became a total abstainer as the only way to avoid addiction, telling Hannah More, 'I can't touch a little, child, therefore I never touch it. Abstinence is as easy to me, as temperance would be difficult'.[26]

Trotter's *Essay ... on Drunkenness* is a landmark in the history of thinking about drunkenness, alcoholism and addiction; yet precisely in which ways and for what reasons remain open to question, for he was probably not quite the pioneer he thought himself to be. (One wonders why he nowhere refers to the discussions of the problem by Cheyne, Mandeville, Lettsom, Rush and others.) The remainder of this introductory essay will seek to ascertain the precise contribution made by Trotter. It will not principally address the rather Whiggish issue of priority (was Trotter the first to adumbrate the modern idea of alcoholism?). Instead, it will aim to recapture exactly which elements of drunkenness fascinated Trotter as a well-trained, experienced and humane practitioner, and how he viewed drunkenness as a medico-social problem and a therapeutic challenge. It is first relevant to sketch his life.

Introduction by Roy Porter

The Life of Thomas Trotter, 1760–1832

We do not know whether Trotter accentuated or tried to suppress his Scottishness, but the fact that he was born in Scotland – at Melrose in Roxburghshire in 1760 – was of immense importance in shaping his career and attitudes.[27] A baker's son – he sprang from the same class of society as the Hunter brothers – Trotter went off at the age of seventeen to Edinburgh University to study medicine. It is known that he took Alexander Monro Secundus's class in anatomy and surgery. After two years he left, perhaps out of ambition, perhaps from poverty, and elected one of the classic career options open to the young Scottish medical lad of parts: he became a surgeon's mate in the Navy.

The War of American Independence was then at its height, and Trotter almost immediately found himself on active service aboard the *Berwick* bound for the Caribbean. Caught in a dreadful hurricane in which he lost his medicine chest, the ship limped back to England with a crew severely stricken with scurvy and dysentery (Trotter himself suffered badly from the latter). This youthful experience undoubtedly made a profound impact upon him. Throughout his naval career, improving the health of sailors was to be his great priority. It was, in any case, as he noted, a matter of military prudence: as he was to discover, the Royal Navy's victories at sea owed much to the fact that the French were saddled with sick crews. This initial trip also fixed his lifelong concern with scurvy, which he first discussed in print in his *Observations on the Scurvy* (1786).

Trotter saw further active service, receiving public thanks for his exemplary treatment of the wounded at the Battle of Dogger Bank in 1781, and being promoted to the rank of surgeon in the next year. At the close of the war in 1783, Trotter found himself one of those surgeons unfortunate enough not to be kept on at half pay. He took employment instead on a Liverpool slave ship, the *Brookes*. It proved another harrowing experience. The inhumanities of the slave trade appalled him, and he discovered that his elementary medical advice (for instance, for purchasing such antiscorbutics as fresh vegetables and fruit) was ignored by the callous and bigoted master, interested in nothing but economy. Trotter's early experiences taught him two lessons. First, that the difference between a healthy ship and a disastrously disease-ridden one lay in the dedication and authority of the surgeon; and second, that immense resistance was to be expected from the traditionalism, stupidity or parsimony of the officer class.

Trotter next practised briefly at Wooler in Northumberland, before returning to Edinburgh, where he attended the lectures of William Cullen, Francis Home, James Gregory and Daniel Rutherford, and, under the imprimatur of James Gregory and the encouragement of Dr Charles Webster, wrote his MD dissertation, *De Ebrietate, Eiusque Effectibus in Corpus Humanum* (1788).[28] It was apparently warmly received by Cullen. Little is known in any detail about Trotter's activities during his two spells in Edinburgh. It is clear, however, that he became caught up in the controversies surrounding John Brown and his Brunonian doctrines. In both the *De Ebrietate* and in the later *Essay ... on Drunkenness*, Trotter drew on the Brunonian concept of excitation, while taking issue with the Brunonians for holding too simplistic a vision of health as the mid-point between extreme sthenic and asthenic conditions.[29]

On leaving Edinburgh, Trotter then resumed his career in the Navy medical service. Armed with his MD, he now became a naval physician, being appointed to the *Barfleur* in 1788. He quickly attracted notice as an active and highly conscientious man, not afraid to voice strong views on the vital importance of cleanliness, ventilation and diet for maintaining health aboard ship. From 1793 to 1794 he served as second physician at Haslar, the vast naval hospital – it held up to 2,000 patients – just outside Portsmouth. Without being fixated upon pet theories, Trotter proved energetic in striving for improvements, in particular seeking to better the quality of nursing care, spelling out his ideas in *Remarks on the Establishment of the Naval Hospitals with Hints for their Improvement* (1795). Even so, the resistance his agitations met grieved him. Although the reforms he aimed to introduce were relatively uncontroversial – such as a suite of baths and a vegetable garden – they met with mere inertia.

In 1794 Trotter was promoted to his highest appointment, physician to the Channel Fleet under Lord Howe, with whom he enjoyed cordial relations. His massive three-volume *Medicina Nautica: An Essay on the Diseases of Seamen*, published in 1797, 1799 and 1803, a medical history of the Channel Fleet from 1794 to 1802, affords a fascinating glimpse of his endeavours.[30] He encouraged record-keeping amongst the ships' surgeons, and placed great faith in the value in tabulating data of epidemics, their duration, severity and outcome. He agitated for practical improvements in operating facilities and recovery beds, preferring to tend sailors aboard ship than to transfer them to hospitals on shore. Not least, he campaigned to raise the pay and conditions of naval surgeons.

Trotter always affected to despise theory and trust to experience. Yet he was no blind empiricist. In assessing the aetiology of diseases aboard ship, he recognized a certain truth in the miasmatic theory: foul air and lack of ventilation bred diseases. Yet some diseases were clearly spread by contagion, smallpox in particular. For that reason, he championed inoculation throughout the navy, and quickly became one of the most ardent supporters of Jennerian vaccination (the *Essay ... on Drunkenness* was to be dedicated to Jenner, and they became friendly correspondents).[31] Though perhaps curiously ambivalent towards James Lind (of Lind's methods with scurvy, he wrote, 'the plain truth is, his method of cure was imperfect', and he disapproved of Lind's passion for fumigation), Trotter was a lifelong propagandist for the value of citrus fruits, lemons above all, and of fresh vegetables in preventing and treating scurvy; and he was fond of picturing himself, as physician to the fleet, personally scouring the markets and nurseries in and around ports, buying up the choicest apples and onions for his crews. Trotter was not specially concerned with the theoretical reasons why fruit and vegetables proved efficacious antiscorbutics, though in his *Medical and Chemical Essays* (1795), not one of his more successful works, he offered reasons for regarding them, in line with the new Lavoisierian chemistry, and particularly following Beddoes's pneumatic experiments, as providing the blood with an acidifying principle, oxygen being the principle of fighting disease.[32]

Trotter suffered a hernia in 1795, and this perhaps precipitated the early end to his naval career in 1802. On leaving the service, he was awarded no special honours or recognition, and not a penny above his regular pension of £200 p.a. His later writings indicate that he took this as an affront, believing that this rather shoddy treatment was the reward for his tireless badgering of the naval powers-that-be on behalf of crews and surgeons. The *Medica Nautica* may in part be read as a retrospective self-vindication, indicting the supineness of his naval superiors and of such fashionable naval physicians as Sir Gilbert Blane; and the *Essay ... on Drunkenness* likewise abounds with barbs against the complacency of those whose duty was to improve the sailor's lot, as well as celebrating his own achievements, as for example in securing a reduction of the number of gin shops in Plymouth from 300 to 100.[33]

Just turned forty, Trotter chose to settle as a medical practitioner in Newcastle, an obvious choice for a seafaring man, though an ambitious ex-physician to the fleet might have been expected to set up in London. In 1810, on the death of his first wife, he remarried. He played an active part in the intellectual and cultural life of the town, being prominent in the Literary and Philosophical Society and contributing to the local newspapers and journals. His interests were both literary and scientific. He published a play, *The Noble Foundling*, in 1812, and a volume of poems, *Sea Weeds: Poems Written on Various Occasions, Chiefly During a Naval Life*, in 1829. But he also became embroiled in the controversy over the prevention of gas explosions in the deep pits of the Northumberland and Durham coalfields. As set out in his *A Proposal for Destroying the Fire and Choak-damp of Coal Mines* (1805), Trotter's solution lay in the use of an effective ventilation system – a view which surely reflects his years of experience in keeping ships' holds salubrious.

For one who had risen to become chief naval physician, and who was to publish influential works in his forties, relatively little is known of the last twenty-five years of Trotter's life. He continued as a medical practitioner in Newcastle till he was in his mid-sixties. Retiring from practice in 1827, he moved to a small estate in his native Roxburghshire, then briefly to Edinburgh, before finally returning to Newcastle, where he died on 5 September 1832. The last quarter century of his life brought no further medical or scientific publications.

Trotter's three chief productions all appeared around mid-life. These were the *Medicina Nautica* (1797–9), the summation of his experience in the navy, which will not be further discussed; the *Essay ... on Drunkenness* (1804), which will be analysed below; and the *View of the Nervous Temperament* (1807). This was in many respects Trotter's most wide-ranging and intellectually ambitious medical work – it is approximately twice as long as the *Essay ... on Drunkenness* – constituting an attempt to diagnose the characteristic sicknesses of the age, indeed, more specifically, to pinpoint precisely how the degeneracy of modern society was itself creating a proclivity towards sickness. The *View of the Nervous Temperament* has been neglected. I shall attempt to show below how a grasp of its key ideas is vital to an understanding of Trotter's project in the *Essay . . . on Drunkenness*.

The *Essay . . . on Drunkenness*

Trotter's *Essay . . . on Drunkenness* (1804) is a quite complex literary production. For one thing, it stands in a rather unusual relationship to his Edinburgh University MD dissertation, *De Ebrietate* (1788). Trotter quotes from his MD in the original Latin,[34] presumably as a way of establishing the temporal priority of his ideas about the diseases of drink. Yet he also treats the *De Ebrietate* as the first edition of the work of which the *Essay . . . on Drunkenness* is the 'second' ('corrected and enlarged'). Thus we encounter the peculiar situation of an author quoting from the first edition of his own work in the second edition! Trotter awkwardly terms his *Essay* a 'comment' on his MD thesis.

This is just one sign amongst many that the *Essay . . . on Drunkenness* was having to serve a plurality of purposes. After having spent twenty years in His Majesty's Service, Trotter had newly set up as a physician in civilian life. Though his choice of Newcastle may possibly mark a decision for relative retirement, the fact that he was keen to make a name for himself as a medical author also suggests ambition. Citing his pioneering MD thesis may well have been part of a strategy for establishing his credentials within the medical community as an expert of long-standing upon inebriation.

Yet all the signs are that he was not primarily, or at least not solely, targeting the *Essay* at a professional, medical readership. Written in an entertaining and often personal style, and laced with anecdotes and asides, the work is far from being a dry handbook or technical treatise on habitual drunkenness, methodically detailing its diagnosis and treatment, and listing clinical case histories and therapeutics. For one thing, as already mentioned, Trotter uses it as a vehicle to hit back against the 'torpid indifference' of the naval authorities – sardonically referring in his dedication to Jenner to

'my present obscurity'.[35] For another, he was clearly putting himself through his paces as a man of letters – an ambition eventually
manifesting itself in his plays and verse: several chapters begin with
epigraphs from Shakespeare, and extracts from Horace, Virgil,
James Thomson, Robert Burton and other literary lions are spliced
into the text. It is noticeable that Trotter offers as his prime depic-
tion of the characteristics of intoxication Falstaff's paean to the
qualities of a 'good sherries sack'.[36]

Yet Trotter's work is far from being 'merely' a literary essay; nor
is it intended to add to the genre of do-it-yourself domestic health-
care books written primarily for the laity, for unlike these, Trotter
does not dole out platitudinous advice upon the virtues of temperance. It would also be misleading to suggest that his *Essay* is just a
mishmash, falling between many different stools. Perhaps the indications that Trotter had several different purposes in mind confirms
that, as he claimed, he was indeed initiating a genre of writing about
drunkenness, rather than contributing to a well-worn tradition.

Above all, Trotter wants the medical identity of his monograph
to be established beyond dispute. It is surely significant that he
chooses to dedicate it to 'Dr Jenner', thereby, by implication at
least, playing off the medical benefactor of mankind against the
Admiralty top brass whom he might he expected to have sought as
patrons. He also takes an early opportunity of slighting the efforts
of the 'priesthood' and the 'moralist' to rectify drunkenness: though
such lay people have 'meant well', in the event they have done little
good, because the key medical aspect – 'the physical influence of
custom, confirmed into habit, interwoven with the actions of our
sentient system, and reacting on our mental part' – has 'been entirely
forgotten'. Drunkenness must be recognized as the province of the
'discerning physician'.[37] And in pursuit of this he chooses to give
his book a medical structure, or, as he puts it, 'to treat my subject
philosophically'.[38]

The first chapter concerns itself with the 'Definition of Drunkenness', and opens with the challenging and programmatic character-
ization of drunkenness as 'strictly speaking ... a disease'.[39] We
must, of course, be wary of reading too much into this contention;
for to a practitioner trained in the eighteenth century, the term
'disease' still carried general connotations of 'dis-ease', disorder or
distemper, rather than the very specific implications – the notion of

a disease as a distinct ontological entity, a *vera causa* – later to become common in the age of bacteriology and germ theory.[40] Trotter's tactical aim was less to make the fine distinction between drunkenness as 'disease' and drunkenness as symptom, than to assert categorically that drunkenness fell within the medical domain.

As he goes on to explain, to label drunkenness a disease is a way of identifying it as equivalent in status to other disease entities such as delirium, apoplexy or coma, with which of course it shares symptoms and to which it commonly leads.[41] Thus, in Trotter's definition, drunkenness is specified as the disease consequent upon 'immoderate use of vinous liquors', producing the symptoms of 'imbecility of intellect, erroneous judgment, violent emotions and loss of sense and motion'.[42] Addressing the eminent professor, William Cullen's nosology, Trotter places drunkenness within the class of the *Vesaniae*, i.e., the species of insanity; within this category it has the closest affinities to *amentia* (idiotism), *insania*, and *mania* though *melancholia* is itself often the consequence of habitual intoxication.[43]

Having arrived at his medical definition of drunkenness, Trotter proceeds in his second chapter to investigate its 'phenomena and symptoms'. The initial effects of alcohol – the desired end of drinking – are to suffuse heat, stimulus, ardour, vigour; but when continued beyond moderation there follows a descent from stimulus to 'indirect debility', 'from pleasure to pain, from the purest perceptions of intellect to the last confusion of thought', which 'ends, by bringing [man] to a level with the brutes'.[44] Trotter details the symptoms of common drunkenness ('the countenance looks swollen and inflamed, the eyes start and glare, vision is double', he writes, citing Boissier de Sauvages),[45] but also describes the acute 'paroxysm', which triggers fever, delirium, apoplexy and even death. Therein lies the paradox at the heart of 'vinolency' (apparently an archaic term, revived by Trotter): prolonged potations prove counter-productive. Moreover, its use as a stimulant is subject to the law of diminishing returns: ever greater quantities are successively needed to induce identical effects: 'in short', states Trotter in a comment that is more than just a truism, 'like all human enjoyments, the exhilarating powers of wine lose their fine zest and high relish, by being too frequently indulged'.[46]

Having defined drunkenness and examined its phenomena and effects, Trotter proceeds, in chapter III, to explore the powers of alcohol upon the animal economy: through what chemical and vital processes does it produce its effects? To resolve this, Trotter feels obliged to pose a much wider question, not confined to alcoholic beverages but encompassing the entire range of 'narcotics' – in particular opium, bangue, hyosciamus (henbane), nicotiana and so forth. Should alcohol and other such substances be principally regarded as 'sedatives'? Or should they rather be treated – as the Brunonian school insisted – primarily and essentially as 'stimulant and exciting', being only 'indirectly sedatives', once their stimulating power had been exhausted?[47] Focusing upon the effects of opium, used medically and recreationally, Trotter contends that the latter is evidently the correct reading – after all, he stresses, no physician would prescribe opium for inflammatory or sthenic diseases such as pneumonia, which clearly require sedative treatment. Hence, Trotter concludes, 'all narcotics have more or less the same effect'.[48]

It may seem that Trotter is here making heavy weather of an obvious empirical fact: that vinous spirits are a stimulant. But his ploy was designed to secure two larger points. On the one hand, he was aiming to establish the affinity between consuming alcohol and recourse to a multitude of other stimulants, all seen as manifestations of a common sociopathology – a point to which I shall return later. On the other, by assimilating drinking within the use of 'narcotics' in general, he sought to provide a general formulaic answer to the problem of the physiological effects of alcohol. What is the nature of the 'operation of vinous spirit on the body'? It is, he can now answer, 'intoxicating'.[49]

Trotter was aware of the verbal sleight of hand involved in this solution, to which he presumably resorted for want of any detailed experimental physiological studies of the kind performed later in the nineteenth century. Possibly in a gesture of self-exculpatory bravado for the rather Molièrian quality of the solution (alcohol makes people drunk because it is intoxicating), Trotter waves further inquiry aside as pointless: it is beyond our power to trace the pathways through which alcohol affects the fibres, nerves and brain, and 'it would be an endless digression, and very little useful to the present investigation, to detail the various theories and conjectures of physicians and metaphysicians on the connection between body and mind'.[50]

Instead, Trotter pursues some of the side-effects of intoxication. Drunkenness suspends or distorts many regular vital processes and sensory-motor chains. It has been alleged to offer protection against certain contagions (Trotter is non-committal); it certainly provides a surprising immunity against extreme cold and other painful sensations; and not least it disorientates the senses, allowing Trotter to quote some entertaining anecdotes out of Burton's *Anatomy of Melancholy* (1621) concerning drunkards' delusions.[51]

Alongside its 'intoxicating' principle of action, alcohol also possesses a 'chemical' power, which he regards, in a manner apparently indebted to Beddoes, as intimately connected with deoxygenation of the blood. Trotter devotes full thirty pages of his text to exploring one particular manifestation of the chemical transformations of chronic drunkenness: spontaneous combustion, or, as he defines it, 'the burning of the human body without the contact of any substance in a state of ignition'.[52] He adduces a handful of apparently well-documented examples – mostly fat old sottish women – in which, as was said, the consequence of protracted heavy spirit-drinking was to turn the body fibres and fat into a kind of highly combustible fuel. Possibly with the aid of an initial spark from a pipe, such people, their bodies literally soaked and pickled, had caught fire and insensibly burned to death in their sleep. Trotter acknowledges the bizarreness of these tales, but is disposed to accept them, believing them well-authenticated.[53] They clearly support his more general proposition, that man is a creature comprehensively changed, morally and physically, by his mode of living – or, as he might have said, man is what he drinks. They also, of course, provide the most awful warning:[54] 'May men never forget that the vine sometimes produces very bitter fruit, – disease, pain, repentance, and DEATH!'

But burning to death is not the only dire fate awaiting the drunkard, and Trotter devotes his fourth chapter to an exposition of the spectrum of diseases which 'temulency' brings on. These divide into two kinds; on the one hand, those acute disorders specifically triggered while in a state of high inebriation – and here apoplexy is the chief,[55] though epilepsy, hysterics and convulsions are also discussed.[56] On the other, those which follow from 'habitual intoxication'. These include inflammatory diseases (brain-fever, pleurisy, rheumatism, and assorted inflammation of the stomach and the bowels),[57] ophthalmia,[58] carbuncles,[59] hepatitis,[60] gout,[61] schirrus,[62] jaundice,[63] dyspepsia,[64] dropsy,[65] tabes and other forms of emaciation,[66] palpitations,[67] diabetes,[68] palsy,[69] ulcers,[70] madness,[71] melancholy,[72] impotence,[73] and premature old age.[74]

Because, one imagines, of his unequalled experience of seeing the physical decline and fall of heavy drinkers in the Navy, Trotter is insistent upon the prime role played by excessive drinking in the aetiology of all such serious diseases. Discussing 'dropsies, apoplexies, palsies, &c.' he comments, 'we must look to hard drinking as the principal agent in bringing on these maladies'.[75] Not least, Trotter stresses, drunkards may communicate their disorders to their children, primarily through the mother's milk, which will all too readily set the baby off on the road to ruin.[76]

So where lies the solution? In chapter V ('The Method of Correcting the Habit of Drunkenness, and of Treating the Drunken Paroxysm') Trotter addresses himself to counter-measures. It is perhaps the most radical and original section in the whole work. Trotter abstains from droning the customary warning sermon, nor does he pretend that he has in his bag a surefire medical therapeutic – still less a nostrum – to redeem addicts. Instead his approach is to characterise alcohol-dependency as integral to, and one element of many within, a wider contemporary problem of addiction to stimulants and narcotics. In his view, habitual drinking will be misunderstood unless contextualized alongside the rampantly rising consumption of opiates, tea, coffee, cordials, and (not least) medicines, and the development of other harmful habits. To concentrate upon the individual sot would be to commit the error of scapegoating; the problem was much wider, and would be intelligible only within the framework of what we might anachronistically call a comprehensive historical sociology of health and sickness.

Within the confines of a single chapter, Trotter can sketch in this framework only suggestively, merely through a variety of examples and anecdotes. The Ancients, he tells us, guarded themselves effectively against this horrid habit of intoxication; under one of Solon's laws, the Athenians put drunken magistrates to death; to excite horror of tipsiness amongst their children, the Spartans exposed drunken slaves before them; 'amongst the Romans, the vice was odious: the whole history of this republic does not mention such a phrase, as a habit of intoxication'.[77]

Nowadays, by contrast, he argues it is thought manly rather than shameful to have a name for being a heavy drinker, and – wagging a disapproving finger at politicians such as Fox and Pitt – in these degenerate times it is even thought proper that a statesman should be a three-bottle man.[78] Nor, Trotter implied, were the ladies any better, for in different ways they were no less addicted – albeit often secretively – to their brandy-based cordials, opiates and laudanum, to say nothing of their countless dishes of intoxicating hyson tea.[79] So-called civilized Christians dub Red Indians and similar people barbarians, yet the Cherokees have absolutely prohibited the use of hard liquor;[80] and so forth.

It is easy to pick up the thread of the argument implied in such disparate remarks. But there is no need to strain at these hints, because Trotter spelt out his case more systematically and lengthily in his *View of the Nervous Temperament*, which can profitably be read as an extended gloss upon, and contextualization of, the *Essay ... on Drunkenness*.

Drunkenness and the Nervous Temperament

The *View of the Nervous Temperament* engages with the debate over the gains and losses of man's emergence from 'rudeness to refinement' – Trotter himself picks up that famous phrase – conducted throughout the Enlightenment, above all by Montesquieu and Rousseau in France and by Adam Ferguson, Adam Smith and John Millar in Scotland.[81] Such 'conjectural historians', or philosophical anthropologists, could broadly agree that history showed epochal transformations of human culture: man had developed the useful and the fine arts, and maximized his control over Nature; with greater technical and scientific powers, economic progress had multiplied wealth and leisure; social organization had become more sophisticated, manners and morals had grown more polite, refined and sensitive. Modern society seemed to abound in affluence, comforts and individual liberty, in enticing opportunities and higher expectations.

What was fundamentally disputed, however, was the deeper

meaning of these developments for human nature and happiness, for man's real well-being, psychic and physical. Optimists argued that as a result of these advances man now lived in a safer, securer, more healthy environment, and could exercise greater control over his destiny. Education, urbanity and refinement, had increased his potential for happiness, and economic and technological progress had extended his capacity to realise that potential. Thus, at the close of the third volume of his *Decline and Fall of the Roman Empire*, Edward Gibbon could claim along these lines, with a flourish tinged with a hint of scepticism, that 'every age of the world has increased, and still increases, the real wealth, the happiness, the knowledge, and perhaps the virtue, of the human race'.[82]

Trotter read Gibbon,[83] but advanced a clean contrary interpretation of the implications of this epochal transition. In a way more reminiscent of Rousseau, Trotter looked back to the more basic civilizations of Antiquity, and even to the barbarians as portrayed by Tacitus, and saw in them peoples marked by a noble 'simplicity'.[84] They were sturdy, independent and tough; they suffered few ills, precisely because they had few needs: 'where the savage feels one want, the civilized being has a thousand'.[85] It might be admitted of the 'primitive', Trotter conceded, that 'his enjoyments are limited'; nevertheless 'his cares, his pains, and his diseases are few'.[86]

In Trotter's evaluation, the march of civilization, with its attendant claustrophobic urbanization, indoors existence, 'refined life',[87] and sedentary occupations (or none at all!)[88] has proved little more than the advance of discontents, generated by spiralling wants, opportunities and desires. The tide of progress has fermented a spirit of inquietude, a restless, insatiable quest for new experiences, new gratifications, new excitements. Greater wealth has brought idleness, indolence and consequent 'low spirits';[89] these in turn have spurred fresh cravings for 'debilitating pleasures'[90] and 'excessive stimuli'.[91] Similarly, indulgence in luxury begat the evils of excess,[92] and the cultivation of subtler tastes and exquisite sensitivities brought with them increased susceptibilities to pain.

By consequence, alongside cravings for novel stimuli, fresh needs sprang up for sedatives, to deaden the pains of the discontents of civilization – not least that 'hypochondriacism' resulting from a combination of unhealthy life-styles and ultra-febrile imagination.[93] The civilizing process thus created insatiable needs for both 'inordinate stimulation'[94] and for narcotics, all fired by the allure of the new and the empire of fashion. More specifically, the artifices of modish living – over-sophisticated diet, gluttony,[95] stifling rooms, pernicious fashions such as tight-laced corsets, late rising, lack of exercise and so forth – necessarily bred ill-health and disease, and so led automatically (given the new supersensitivity to pain) to the swallowing of ever greater quantities of medicines; and because so many of these were both harmful and addictive, they in turn further destroyed the stomach and the nerves, causing fresh sickness, and so induced a descending spiral of yet more medicines to rectify the iatrogenic ailments.

All in all, judged Trotter, the so-called growth of freedom in modern society was all illusory. Pleasures rapidly wore out and trapped the voluptuary on a treadmill, for – to return to a sentiment expressed in the *Essay ... on Drunkenness* – 'the exhilarating powers ... lose their fine zest and high relish, by being too frequently indulged'.[96] Thus modern man was enslaving himself to his own insatiable imagination, wants and expectations, to his vices and his self-created physical and mental weaknesses. We had degenerated, bemoaned Trotter, into a 'nation of slaves'.[97] In its currently morbid manifestations civilization was itself a mode of disease.

So civilized man grew unhealthy, suffering from that very 'nervous temperament' which the civilizing process had created. To revive his jaded appetites he resorted to such stimuli as ardent spirits; to ease his pains and deaden his jangled nerves, he swallowed sedatives; all these in turn only gave new twists to the screws of sickness. Medicines proper had the same deplorable effects. And all the while, Trotter emphasized, implicitly drawing upon Lockean associationist theories of the formation of habit and character through education and environment, these pathological facets of civilization were actually becoming ingrained within human nature itself, embossed upon the collective mind and passed down from generation to generation. For human nature was not a fixed entity, but the product of self-development. And civilized man, a delicate, hothouse plant, was above all a 'creature of habit'.[98] In so far as he was a victim of the 'nervous temperament', this was precisely because he was the 'creator of his own temperament'.[99] As Trotter emphasized in his *Essay*, 'in the present stage of society, human kind are almost taken out of the hands of Nature; and a custom called *fashion* ... now rules everything'.[100]

In individual, society, and race, the disposition to drunkenness was both a symptom and a spur within this process. The craving for drink was itself a mark of an effeminate, decadent stage, for 'natural appetite requires no such stimulants'.[101] Trotter was not such a primitivist as to debar stimulants entirely. But most – such as ardent spirits and hyson tea – he believed were essentially harmful; and he deplored the fact that stimulants such as wine, which were safe if deployed wisely, had been turned into necessities, and that such substances as soda water, which ought to be used strictly medicinally, had become habitual beverages. Times were bad when opium, God's greatest gift to the physician for the relief of acute pain, had become an item in every fashionable lady's reticule in the form of the laudanum phial.[102]

Thus, in both the individual and in the social macrocosm, a descending spiral was in motion. Drawing upon the Brunonian analysis of excitability, Trotter asserted that each dose of artificial stimulant produced the required sensations, but only temporarily, and their powers to excite were quickly exhausted. They were then consumed in ever larger quantities, greater concentrations, or in adulterated forms – and here Trotter was particularly severe on the adulterating practices of the great brewers.[103] Finally, more potent stimulants had to be found. Time was when the rich had satisfied their cravings in wine; now, enervated by 'luxury and refinement'[104] and racked by 'diseased sensibility',[105] they had taken to fortified liquors such as port and brandy. Formerly the poor had quaffed their ale; now they downed rum and gin, or, no less perniciously, ales adulterated by unscrupulous brewers who added addictive bitters and even opiates.

Overall then, 'polished society' was so acting as to 'bring on its own dotage' and 'dig its own grave'.[106] There was nothing fundamentally original in Trotter's interpretation of how the transition from 'rudeness to refinement'[107] had in reality proved disastrous for human nature. Many other critics looked back to a golden age when life was simpler, healthier, happier. Indeed such advocacy of plain living was quite common amongst doctors, from George Cheyne's *English Malady*, which urged a return to grains and milk, through to the late eighteenth-century sex therapist, James Graham, who indicted oversophisticated civilization of causing impotence and depopulation, demanding an end to alcohol consumption and a return to water.[108] Cheyne had suggested that perhaps a third of all the diseases of 'people of condition' were nervous; Trotter, probably echoing him, judged that such diseases constituted no less than two-thirds of all modern disorders.[109]

Though Trotter's account of the diseases of civilization was not, strictly speaking, original, what makes his formulation of these ideas particularly telling is his stress on the symbiosis of physical and psychological dependency in the individual (increasingly hooked on his stimulants, be they alcohol or medicines), and indeed in that 'a creature of habit and imitation',[110] civilized man at large, was 'wallowing in wealth and rioting in indulgence',[111] enslaved to the tyranny of fashion, sensation, and novelty. Physical stimuli, such as alcohol, made their mark upon the senses; these in turn registered their effects upon the nervous system, producing the 'nervous temperament'; this temperament affected the psyche; and in turn the mind begat imagined desires which set off new chains of cravings. Thus Trotter could ask, rhetorically:[112] 'Are not habits of drunkenness more often produced by mental affections than corporeal diseases? I apprehend few people will doubt the truth of this.' Convinced thus of this psychological enslavement, it was natural that Trotter should be the first analyst clearly to formulate the idea of habitual drunkenness as a mental illness, for in his view it was sustained by a wider historical process of the corruption of the civilized mind.

Trotter was never an out-and-out primitivist, advocating a return to Nature, as Rousseau seemed in some of his more provocative pronouncements. Indeed, he thought that certain pockets of hardy manhood still survived relatively uncorrupted. A well-disciplined British warship, manned by doughty tars and commanded by conscientious officers, was one exception, and he was confident that Britain would defeat Napoleon, for the process of cultural decadence, the evolution of the nervous temperament, had proceeded less in Britain than in effeminate France.[113] Hence he was not merely a *laudator temporis acti*, and it was the abuses of civilization, not civilization itself, which he deplored. He did not call for the total abandonment of medicine or alcohol, nor did he envisage the state passing any general liquor laws. What he recommended, rather, was the time-honoured regime of moderation.

In respect of alcohol, he was guided largely by considerations of health. No healthy young man should require the stimulus of vinous spirits. At the age of forty, a man might avail himself of the cheering and cordial virtues of good wine to the extent of two glasses a day; at fifty, that might be extended to four, and at sixty to six. On this Trotter cited Luigi Cornaro, the renowned Venetian writer on longevity who had lived to well over a hundred on such a regime.[114] The pursuit of 'temperance' in the traditional sense – i.e., moderation – would curb the insensate lust for sensation fired by the nervous temperament.

But were remedies to hand in the case of the individual sufferer? For those actually in the throes of the drunken paroxysm, Trotter suggested the standard drastic countermeasures to prevent possibly fatal apoplexy, above all, emetics and clysters. The habitual drunkard was a different problem. For those 'addicted to ebriety',[115] pursuit of a sensible regimen of 'plain diet and water'[116] was of course vital; and such expedients as visits to Bath might be useful. But on one point Trotter was insistent. Precisely because habitual drunkenness was a disease of the mind, it must be cured not by drugs, but by mental discipline: 'it is in vain to expect a cure from articles of medicine. The habit of drinking must cease, and moral arguments ... must be speedily employed'.[117] This would require the strict 'ascendency' of the physician over his wayward and morally perverse patient – Trotter's formulation here echoes the 'moral management' techniques prominent in contemporary psychiatry.[118]

Not least, because habitual drunkenness was a mental disorder, successful cures required that drinking should stop 'at once', rather than by gradual stages: it must be marked by an act of will. Trotter surveyed the strategems widely advocated to wean sots off drink gradually – e.g., Lettsom's ruse of putting a drop of sealing-wax in the drunkard's glass each day, so as slowly and insensibly to reduce his intake.[119] Trotter dismissed such ploys as 'childish' and psychologically stupid. The drunkard, 'addicted to the bottle',[120] would naturally drink a little, feel good on it, and persuade himself it was safe to take a little more. Only a sudden, decisive, complete break would work. It had all to be done 'at once'.[121]

Conclusion

At first glance, Trotter's *Essay ... on Drunkenness* may appear rather a strange book, both perceptive and pioneering, with its stress upon habitual drunkenness as a disease, indeed a disease of the mind, yet puzzlingly anecdotal, short of specific clinical evidence, case studies and therapeutic experiments. It is certainly not a work in the mould of nineteenth century psychiatric discussions of alcoholism, typically focused upon the data of alienism as taken from the lunatic asylum – an institution Trotter does not even mention. The proper integrity is, however, restored to his work if it is seen, in tandem with the *View of the Nervous Temperament*, in the light of the emphasis placed by Scottish medicine, in particular Cullen's school, upon the overwhelming importance of the nervous system (and thus of neurosis), and upon the role played by nervous organization in the interplay of mind and body, consciousness and action. Trotter set this insight within the framework of a late Enlightenment historical sociology of the evolution of human wants – and discontents. Drawing upon a tradition of cultural criticism, he viewed the very civilizing process itself, with its quest for stimulus and its cultivation of refined sensibility, as uncorking a magnum of evils. Trotter made a pioneering contribution to the understanding of alcoholism. To understand this, it must be located in its historical context.

Notes

1. For Boswell see K. B. Rix (1975), 'James Boswell (1740–1795): "No Man is More Easily Hurt With Wine than I Am"', *Journal of Alcoholism*, 10: 73–7; for a general and rather anecdotal account of heavy drinking habits see A. L. Simon (1926) *Bottlescrew Days. Wine Drinking in England During the Eighteenth Century*, London: Duckworth.

2. For the place of drinking within pre-industrial society, see J. A. Spring and D. H. Buss, 'Three Centuries of Alcohol in the British Diet', *Nature*, 219 (1977): 567–72; M. M. Glatt, 'The English Drink Problem: its Rise and Decline Through the Ages', *The British Journal of Addiction*, 4 (1958): 51–67; H. G. Graham (1969) *The Social Life of Scotland in the Eighteenth Century*, London: Black; Keith V.

Thomas (1971) *Religion and the Decline of Magic*, London: Weidenfeld & Nicolson: p. 17; P. Clark (1983) *The English Ale House*, London: Longman. Samuel Johnson's views are discussed in J. S. Maddan (1976) 'Samuel Johnson's Alcohol Problem', *Medical History*, 11: 141–5.

3. For Mather see M. Lender (1973), 'Drunkenness as an Offence in Early New England', *Quarterly Journal for Studies in Alcoholism*, 34: 357. For medical approval of drinking see P. Shaw (1724) *The Juice of the Grape; or Wine Preferable to Water*, London: W. Lewis. For religious tolerance see M. Screech (1979) *Rabelais*, London: Duckworth, and Screech (1983) *Montaigne and Melancholy*, London: Duckworth. Thomas Trotter himself complained about the lacing of nostrums with alcohol: see Trotter (1804) *An Essay, Medical, Philosophical, and Chemical, on Drunkenness and its Effects on the Human Body*, London: Longman, Hurst, Rees & Orme. Similar points are made in V. Berridge and G. Edwards (1982) *Opium and the People*, New Haven: Yale University Press.

4. E. L. Bristow (1977) *Vice and Vigilance*, Dublin: Gill & Macmillan; J. Sharpe (1977) 'Crime and Delinquency in an Essex Parish 1640–1660', in J. S. Cockburn (ed.) *Crime in England 1550–1800*, London: Methuen, pp. 90–109; M. J. Ingram, 'Communities and Courts: Law and Disorder in Early Seventeenth Century Wiltshire', in ibid.; pp. 110–34; and, for America, I. Tyrrell (1979) *Sobering Up*, Westport, Conn.: Greenwood Press.

5. For the gin craze see J. Watney (1976) *Mother's Ruin*, London: Peter Owen; D. M. George (1966) *London Life in the Eighteenth Century*, Harmondsworth: Penguin; T. G. Coffey (1966) 'Beer Street: Gin Lane: Some Views of 18th Century Drinking', *Quarterly Journal for the Study of Alcoholism*, 34: 662–92; Lord Kinross (1959) 'Prohibition in Britain', *History Today*, 9: 493–9.

6. See the discussion in P. Mathias (1969) *The Brewing Industry in England 1700–1830*, Cambridge: Cambridge University Press. Trotter's complaints can be found in his *Essay . . . on Drunkenness*, pp. 41f.

7. For the temperance movement see B. Harrison (1971) *Drink and the Victorians*, London: Faber & Faber, and (1963) 'Drunkards and Reformers; Early Victorian Temperance Tracts', *History Today*, 13: 178–85; P. MacCandless (1984) 'Curses of Civilisation; Insanity and Drunkenness in Victorian Britain', *British Journal of Addiction*, 79: 49–58.

8. The views of eighteenth and early nineteenth century mad doctors on drink as a precipitant of insanity are explored in Roy Porter (1987)

Mind Forg'd Manacles. A History of Madness in England from the Restoration to the Regency, London: Athlone Press, pp. 198–201.

9. See the excellent account in W. F. Bynum (1968), 'Chronic Alcoholism in the First Half of the 19th Century', *Bulletin of the History of Medicine* 42: 160–85, esp. p. 162; and John Romano (1941), 'Early Contributions to the Study of *Delirium Tremens*', *Annals of Medical History*, 3: 128–39. For Erasmus Darwin see E. Darwin (1794–6) *Zoonomia; or, the Laws of Organic Life*, 2 vols, London: Johnson. Darwin explicitly termed 'drunkenness' a disease (in his classification it was number I.1.2.2, a disease of 'irritation').

10. Doctors have traditionally seen the advent of medicalization as progress, arguing that the recognition of underlying physical causes for what had traditionally been seen as sins, vices or crimes, freed patients from stigma. See H. W. Haggard and E. M. Jellinick (1942) *Alcohol Explored*, New York: Doubleday & Doran. Critics have argued on the contrary that it forms part of a strategy, conscious or unconscious, of medical imperialism (see T. Szasz (1975) *Ceremonial Chemistry*, London: Routledge & Kegan Paul).

11. I am here indebted to the account in Bynum, op. cit. (note 9).

12. Ibid., pp. 165, 174–5.

13. Ibid., pp. 177–9.

14. See Harrison, *Drink and the Victorians*, op. cit. (note 7), p. 92.

15. Trotter, *Essay ... on Drunkenness* (note 3), p. 3.

16. Ibid., pp. 1, 8.

17. Ibid., pp. 26, 195.

18. Ibid., pp. 1–2.

19. William Buchan (1776) *Domestic Medicine*, London: W. Strahan. For writings about alcoholic drink since Antiquity see J.-C. Sournia (1986) *Histoire de l'Alcoolisme*, Paris: Flammarion.

20. For Rush (1785), see *An Enquiry into the Effects of Spiritous Liquors on the Human Body*, Boston: Thomas & Andrews; J. Hirsch (1949), 'Enlightened Eighteenth Century Views of the Alcohol Problem', *Journal of the History of Medicine*, 4: 230–6; H. G. Levine (1978), 'The Discovery of Addiction: Changing Conceptions of Habitual Drunkenness in America', *Journal of the Study of Alcoholism*, 39: 143–74, and B. Rush (1948), 'Plan for an Asylum for Drunkards to be Called the Sober House. 1810', reprinted in G. W. Corner (ed.) *The Autobiography of Benjamin Rush*, Princeton: Princeton University Press, pp. 354–55.

21. Trotter, *Essay ... on Drunkenness* (note 3), pp. 8, 179. For similar formulations, see ibid., pp. 128, 182 ('the habit of intoxication belongs to the mind'), p. 26 (drunkenness is 'a species of insanity'),

and p. 186 ('are not habits of drunkenness more often produced by mental affections than corporeal diseases?'). For further discussion, see Roy Porter (1985), 'The Drinking Man's Disease: The "Pre-History" of Alcoholism in Georgian Britain', *British Journal of Addiction*, 80: 385–96.

22. J. C. Lettsom (1787) 'Some Remarks on the Effects of Lignum Quassiae Amarae', *Memoirs of the Medical Society of London*, 1: 128–65, esp. 157–8. For Lettsom, see K. J. Rix (1976) 'John Coakley Lettsom and Some of the Effects of Hard Drinking', *Journal of Alcoholism*, 11: 98–113; and compare also A. Fothergill (1796) *An Essay on the Abuse of Spiritous Liquors*, Bath: Cruttwell, p. 19, and Thomas Beddoes (1802) *Hygeia*, 3 vols, Bristol: Phillips, vol. 2, essay 8, pp. 28–90.

23. G. Cheyne (1724) *An Essay of Health and Long Life*, London: G. Strahan, p. 49.

24. Ibid., p. 53.

25. B. Mandeville (1730) *A Treatise of the Hypochondriack and Hysterick Diseases*, London: J. Tonson, pp. 373–4.

26. J. Wain (1980) *Samuel Johnson*, London: Macmillan, p. 240.

27. The best accounts of Trotter's life, from which most of the following details are taken, are Ian Porter (1963), 'Thomas Trotter, M.D., Naval Physician', *Medical History*, 7: 155–64; Sir Humphry Rolleston (1919) 'Thomas Trotter, M.D.', in *Contributions to Medical and Biological Research Dedicated to Sir William Osler, In Honour of His Seventieth Birthday*, by His Pupils and Co-Workers, New York: Hoeber, pp. 153–65 (perceptive yet unreliable on points of detail). Hardly any manuscript material seems to have survived.

28. Thomas Trotter (1788) *De Ebrietate, Eiusque Effectibus in Corpus Humanum*, Edinburgh. A copy of this is to be found in Edinburgh University Library.

29. The most comprehensive recent discussion of the contribution of Brunonianism to late eighteenth century medical debate is to be found in W. F. Bynum and Roy Porter (eds) (1988) *Brunonianism in Britain and Europe*, London: *Medical History* Supplement 8.

30. Copious extracts from these works have been printed, with a brief commentary, in C. Lloyd (ed.) (1965) *The Health of Seamen. Selections from the Works of Dr. James Lind, Sir Gilbert Blane and Dr. Thomas Trotter*, London: The Navy Records Society, pp. 217–316.

31. See Paul Saunders (1982) *Edward Jenner: The Cheltenham Years 1795–1823*, Hanover and London: The University Press of New England, pp. 107, 255.

32. See Kenneth Carpenter (1986) *The History of Scurvy and Vitamin C*, Cambridge: Cambridge University Press.
33. Trotter, *Essay ... on Drunkenness* (note 3), pp. 41, 49.
34. Ibid., p. 187.
35. Ibid., p. 170.
36. Ibid., p. 20.
37. Ibid., p. 3.
38. Ibid., p. 6.
39. Ibid., p. 8.
40. For discussion of this point see O. Temkin, 'The Scientific Approach to Disease: Specific Entity and Individual Sickness', in A. L. Caplan, H. Tristram Engelhardt, jr, and J. J. McCartney (eds) (1981) *Concepts of Health and Disease*, Reading, Mass.: Addison and Wesley, pp. 247–64; C. Rosenberg, 'The Therapeutic Revolution', in M. Vogel and C. Rosenberg (eds) (1979) *The Therapeutic Revolution*, Philadelphia: University of Pennsylvania Press 3–25.
41. Trotter, *Essay ... on Drunkenness* (note 3), p. 8.
42. Ibid., p. 10.
43. Ibid., p. 11.
44. Ibid., p. 16.
45. Ibid., p. 25.
46. Ibid., p. 29.
47. Ibid., p. 33.
48. Ibid., p. 37.
49. Ibid., p. 42.
50. Ibid., p. 42.
51. Ibid., pp. 47ff.
52. Ibid., p. 87.
53. For discussion see John Rathbone Oliver (1936), 'Spontaneous Combustion', *Bulletin of the History of Medicine*, 4: 559–72.
54. Trotter, *Essay ... on Drunkenness* (note 3), p. 93.
55. Ibid., p. 98.
56. Ibid., p. 105.
57. Ibid., p. 109.
58. Ibid., p. 110.
59. Ibid., p. 111.
60. Ibid., p. 113.
61. Ibid., p. 114.
62. Ibid., p. 116.
63. Ibid., p. 117.
64. Ibid., p. 118.
65. Ibid., p. 121.

66. Ibid., p. 122.
67. Ibid., p. 123.
68. Ibid., p. 124.
69. Ibid., p. 126.
70. Ibid., p. 127.
71. Ibid., p. 129: intoxication is a 'temporary madness'.
72. Ibid., p. 132.
73. Ibid., p. 134.
74. Ibid., p. 135.
75. Ibid., p. 139.
76. Ibid., p. 136.
77. Ibid., p. 140.
78. Ibid., p. 165.
79. Ibid., pp. 154, 174.
80. Ibid., p. 141.
81. See Gladys Bryson (1945) *Man and Society: The Scottish Inquiry of The Eighteenth Century*, Princeton: Princeton University Press.
82. Edward Gibbon (n.d.) *The Decline and Fall of the Roman Empire*, J. B. Bury (ed.) London: Methuen, vol. iv, 169.
83. Thomas Trotter (1807) *A View of the Nervous Temperament, A Practical Enquiry into the Increasing Prevalence, Prevention, and Treatment of those Diseases Commonly Called Nervous, Bilious, Stomach and Liver Complaints; Indigestion; Low Spirits; Gout etc.*, London: Longman, Hurst, Rees & Orme, p. 144.
84. Ibid., p. viii.
85. Ibid., p. 220.
86. Ibid., p. 29.
87. Ibid., p. 35.
88. Ibid., p. 22.
89. Ibid., p. 70.
90. Ibid., p. 48.
91. Ibid., p. 142.
92. Ibid., p. 135; for context see J. Sekora (1977) *Luxury*, Baltimore: Johns Hopkins University Press.
93. Trotter, ibid., p. 39.
94. Ibid., p. 31.
95. Ibid., p. 24.
96. Trotter, *Essay ... on Drunkenness* (note 3), p. 29.
97. Trotter, *View of the Nervous Temperament* (note 83), p. xi.
98. Ibid., p. 31.
99. Ibid., p. 34.
100. Trotter, *Essay ... on Drunkenness* (note 3), p. 153.

101. Ibid., p. 155.
102. Ibid., p. 38; Trotter, *View of the Nervous Temperament* (note 83), p. 312.
103. Trotter, *Essay ... on Drunkenness* (note 3), p. 103.
104. Trotter, *View of the Nervous Temperament* (note 83), p. 135.
105. Ibid., p. 90.
106. Ibid., p. 106.
107. Ibid., p. 143.
108. See H. R. Viets (1949), 'George Cheyne, 1673–1743', *Bulletin of the History of Medicine*, 23: 435–52; Roy Porter (1987) *Mind Forg'd Manacles*, pp. 83–85 (see note 8), and (1982) 'The Sexual Politics of James Graham', *British Journal for Eighteenth Century Studies*, 5: 201–6.
109. Trotter, *View of the Nervous Temperament* (note 83), p. viii.
110. Ibid., p. 233.
111. Ibid., p. 257.
112. Trotter, *Essay ... on Drunkenness* (note 3), p. 186.
113. Trotter, *View of the Nervous Temperament* (note 83), p. 153.
114. Trotter, *Essay ... on Drunkenness* (note 3), p. 156.
115. Ibid., p. 170.
116. Ibid., p. 188.
117. Ibid., p. 120.
118. Ibid., p. 179.
119. Ibid., p. 185.
120. Ibid., p. 195.
121. Ibid., p. 182.

APPENDIX 1:
BIBLIOGRAPHY OF THE WRITINGS OF THOMAS TROTTER

Trotter, T. (1786) *Observations on the Scurvy: with a Review of the Theories Lately Advanced on that Disease; and the Opinions of Dr. Milman Refuted From Practice*, Edinburgh: Charles Elliot & J. Robinson. (2nd edn, 1792)

Trotter, T. (1797–99) *Medicina Nautica; an Essay on the Diseases of Seamen; Comprehending the History of Health in His Majesty's Fleet Under . . . Earl Howe (with an Appendix Containing Communications on the New Doctrine of Contagion and Yellow Fever, By American Physicians, etc.)*, 3 vols, London: Cadell & Davies.

Trotter, T. (1800) *Suspiria Oceani: a Monody on the Death of Richard Earl Howe, K.G., Admiral of the Fleet, etc.*, London: J. Hatchard.

Trotter, T. (1804) *An Essay, Medical, Philosophical, and Chemical, on Drunkenness and its Effects on the Human Body*, London: Longman, Hurst, Rees, & Orme, 2nd edn.

Trotter, T. (1807) *A view of the Nervous Temperament; being a Practical Enquiry into the Increasing Prevalence, Prevention, and Treatment of those Diseases Commonly Called Nervous, Bilious, Stomach and Liver Complaints; Indigestion; Low Spirits; Gout, etc.*, London: Longman, Hurst, Rees, & Orme (2nd edn, 1807) [A third edition appeared in 1812].

Trotter, T. (1819) *A Practicable Plan for Manning the Royal Navy, and Preserving our Maritime Ascendency, without Impressment. Addressed to Admiral Lord Viscount Exmouth*, Newcastle and London: Longman, Hurst, Rees, Orme & Brown.

Trotter, T. (1829) *Sea Weeds. Poems Written on Various Occasions, Chiefly During a Naval Life*, London: Longman.

APPENDIX 2: TROTTER'S MD THESIS: *DE EBRIETATE*

In 1788 Trotter defended and published his MD thesis, *De Ebrietate, Eiusque Effectibus in Corpus Humanum*. Typically of Edinburgh MDs of that vintage, it ran to some forty pages, amounting to perhaps about 8,000 words. It was written in a simple, though quite pure, Latin, and liberally sprinkled with quotations from literary sources, both Classical and English.

Although no more than perhaps a tenth as long as the *Essay ... on Drunkenness*, it is quite unambiguously the parent of the longer and later work. The verbal and stylistic similarities are great. For example, the dissertation begins 'Homines semper studiosi voluptatem aegre inter mala recensuerunt quae ab luxuria orta sunt', which, literally translated, becomes the first sentence of the essay ('Mankind, ever in pursuit of pleasure, have reluctantly admitted into the catalogue of their diseases, those evils which were the immediate offspring of their luxuries'). Already in the dissertation Trotter is proposing 'ebrietatem quasi morbum tractare' (to treat drunkenness as a disease). Above all, the structure of the thesis is remarkably repeated in the *Essay*. The thesis moves from 1. definition, 2. symptoms, 3. proximate causes, 4. original causes, to 5. therapeutics; and this ordering of materials is obviously closely reproduced in the later *Essay*, with much the same reliance upon identical authorities such as Cullen, Morgagni and Boissier de Sauvages.

Certain details and anecdotes are present in the earlier work which have disappeared by the latter, not least, reports on drunken sailors on board his first ship, the *Berwick*. But there is very little indication that any of the views embraced in the *De Ebrietate* were later abandoned. Obviously there is much in the *Essay* without equivalent in the thesis, not least the entire discussion on spontaneous combustion. But there is also evidence of a general broadening of interest in the interim. The *Essay* is noteworthy for the scope of Trotter's concern with the problems of habit and habit-forming substances in general, within the context of (a) the analysis of a drug-consuming culture, and (b) the notion that drunkenness is a disease of the mind. Neither of these concerns had been crystallized in the earlier work. Thus it is fair to say that Trotter began with posing drunkenness as a medical problem; only subsequently did he evolve his major insight, the need to investigate the wider problem of habit and addiction as a whole.

AN

ESSAY,

MEDICAL, PHILOSOPHICAL, AND CHEMICAL,

ON

DRUNKENNESS.

Printed by A. Strahan,
Printers-Street.

A N

E S S A Y,

MEDICAL, PHILOSOPHICAL, AND CHEMICAL,

ON

D R U N K E N N E S S,

AND

ITS EFFECTS ON THE HUMAN BODY.

By THOMAS TROTTER, M. D.

LATE PHYSICIAN TO HIS MAJESTY'S FLEET UNDER THE COMMAND
OF ADMIRAL EARL HOWE, K.G.; AND TO THE SQUADRONS
COMMANDED BY ADMIRAL LORD BRIDPORT, K.B. ADMIRAL
EARL ST. VINCENT, K.B. AND THE HONOURABLE
ADMIRAL CORNWALLIS;
MEMBER OF THE ROYAL MEDICAL SOCIETY OF EDINBURGH;
AN HONORARY MEMBER OF THE ROYAL PHYSICAL SOCIETY
OF EDINBURGH, OF THE MEDICAL SOCIETY OF
ABERDEEN, OF THE PHILOSOPHICAL AND
LITERARY SOCIETY OF NEWCASTLE,
&c. &c.

───────────

O ! thou invisible spirit of wine, if thou hast no name to be
known by, let us call thee—Devil.　　　SHAKSPEARE.

───────────

L O N D O N:

PRINTED FOR T. N. LONGMAN, AND O. REES,
PATERNOSTER-ROW.

1804.

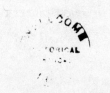

DEDICATION

TO

DR. JENNER.

MY DEAR SIR,

AFTER having addreſſed you on the occaſion of your GREAT DISCOVERY from the firſt medical ſtation in the public ſervice of the country, which I had then the honour to hold, you will be the leſs ſurpriſed to hear from me in my preſent obſcurity. In laying the following Eſſay before the world I feel ſo independent in motive and expectation, that nothing but the patronage of Dr. Jenner can ſatisfy me. I ſhall thus eſcape the common accuſation brought againſt authors of being flatterers. The man whoſe labours go the length of ſaving annually half a million of his fellow-creatures, is as far beyond the ſphere of compliment as he has outſtripped

the

the meafure of human gratitude, and can
need no adulation from my pen. I have,
therefore, to requeft that he will accept of all
that, as a private man, I can offer him, which
is to fay, that, with all fincerity,

I am, my dear Sir,

Your moft faithful friend, and

Moft humble fervant,

Newcaftle-on-Tyne,   T. TROTTER.
    Dec. 26, 1803.

PREFACE.

When I became a candidate for the degree of Doctor of Medicine, in the University of Edinburgh, I was rather anxious that the subject of my Inaugural Diſſertation ſhould be ſomething that had never been noticed by any former graduate. This was a difficult point; for ſcarcely any thing remained that had not been previouſly diſcuſſed. After much conſideration, however, ſeveral objects of inquiry preſented themſelves, and I fixed upon Ebriety. But ſome doubts aroſe in my mind whether ſuch a theſis was proper matter for an academic exerciſe; and as ſoon as I was enabled to put it into a regular form it was ſubmitted to the judgment of the late worthy Dr. Charles Webſter. The doctor was delighted with the work, and gave it as his opinion that it would be highly acceptable to the profeſſors. When my private examinations were finiſhed, it became the taſk of Dr. Gregory, now Profeffor in the Practical Chair, to give it his sanction for being printed. Dr. Gregory perufed it with great pleasure, and encouraged me to think of it as a subject worthy of future investigation. In the public hall my venerable friend and preceptor, Dr. Cullen, was pleased to introduce my examination with some elegant allusions to the thesis; and after a few facetious remarks on the author, in his usual style, commended the design, execution, and importance of the work. I was shortly after this honoured with the thanks of the Humane Society, transmitted to me by Dr. Hawes, the illustrious founder of that institution. Dr. Hawes observed, that, " the investigation of so important an inquiry, in a regular scientific " manner, was never before thought of: it " was a subject left, happily left, to be inge- " niously executed and amplified by Dr. " Trotter."

After such testimonies from men at the summit of the Medical Profession, it became a task of gratitude, as well as duty, with me, to review the Differtation. From 1788 till lately my studies have been entirely occupied

by

by naval affairs; and it is only within thefe few months that I began to compile the following Eſſay, which may be confidered as a comment on the theſis, *De Ebrietate, ejuſque EffeEtLibus in Corpus humanum.* Edin. 1788.

The importance of the undertaking will be generally acknowledged. It is of a nature that muſt intereſt every friend of mankind; and 1 truſt it is demonſtrated in theſe pages the ſhare which the medical profeſſion ought to take in checking the evil habit of intoxication in ſociety. How far I am right in the execution of the plan others muſt decide. I ſhall receive every hint for improvement with much ſatisfaction; and ſhall correct my errors, wherever they may appear, with equal pleaſure.

CONTENTS.

ON DRUNKENNESS, &c.

INTRODUCTION.

—— *Dulce periculum eft,*
O Lenæe ? fequi Deum
Cingentem viridi tempora pampino. Hor.

Mankind, ever in purfuit of pleafure,
have reluctantly admitted into the catalogue
of their difeafes, thofe evils which were the
immediate offspring of their luxuries. Such
a referve is indeed natural to the human
mind : for of all deviations from the paths of
duty, there are none that fo forcibly impeach
their pretenfions to the character of rational
beings as the inordinate ufe of fpirituous liquors. Hence, in the writings of medicine,
we find drunkennefs only curforily mentioned
among the powers that injure health, while
the mode of action is entirely neglected and
left unexplained. This is the more to be
wondered at, as the ftate of ebriety itfelf ex-

hibits

hibits some of the most curious and interesting phænomena that are to be met with in
the history of animated nature. The potent
stimulus of vinous spirit, as if by magical influence, so disturbs, or operates on the animal
functions, that new affections of mind, latent,
or unknown before, are produced; and the
drunkard appears to act the part of a man of
deranged intellect, and altogether foreign to
the usual tenor of his sober reflections.

But a long train of the most dangerous dif-
eases are the certain consequence of habitual
intoxication: the body and mind equally
suffer. Sudden death, apoplexy, palsy, dropsy, madness, and a hideous list of mental dif-
quietudes and nervous failings, prey upon the
shattered frame of the inebriate, and prove
fatal in the end. These sufficiently point out
the subject as highly important in a medical
view, and worthy of the nicest investigation.
But as I have not any precursor in my labours,
nor example in the records of physic, to direct
my steps, I shall need the less apology for the
manner I mean to pursue; and must claim
indulgence where I appear singular in my
method.

Most

Moſt inſtances of caſual or ſudden death, and ſuſpended animation, have obtained rules for recovery ; while the drunkard, expoſed in the ſtreet and highway, or ſtretched in the kennel, has been allowed to periſh, without pity and without aſſiſtance ; as if his crime were inexpiable, and his body infectious to the touch. Our newſpapers give us too fre-quent accounts of this kind. The habit of inebriation, ſo common in ſociety, to be ob-ſerved in all ranks and ſtations of life, and the ſource of inexpreſſible affliction to friends and relatives, has ſeldom been the object of me-dical admonition and practice. The prieſt-hood hath poured forth its anathemas from the pulpit; and the moraliſt, no leſs ſevere, hath declaimed againſt it as a vice degrading to our nature. Both have meant well ; and becomingly oppoſed religious and moral ar-guments to the ſinful indulgence of animal appetite. But the phyſical influence of cuſ-tom, confirmed into habit, interwoven with the actions of our ſentient ſyſtem, and reacting on our mental part, have been entirely for-gotten. The perfect knowledge of thoſe re-mote cauſes which firſt induced the propen-

ſity

sity to vinous liquors, whether they sprung from situation in life, or depended on any peculiar temperament of body, is necessary for conducting the cure. A due acquaintance with the human character will afford much assistance; for the objects of our care are as diversified as the varieties of corporeal structure. Pleasure, on one hand, presents the poisonous bowl: low spirits, on the other, call for the cheering draught. There business and the duties of office have plunged one man into frequent hard drinking; while cares and misfortunes have goaded on another. The soldier and the sailor get drunk while narrating the dangers of the battle and the storm: the huntsman and the jockey, by describing the joys of the chace and course. Here genius and talent are levelled with the dust, in trying to forget, in wine, the outrages of fortune, and the ingratitude of the world; while more ponderous and stupid mortals, in attempting to seek in the bottle the feelings and sentiments of exalted beings, gravitate to their original clay, or sink deeper into their parent mud.

In

In treating thefe various defcriptions of perfons and characters, it will readily appear to a difcerning phyfician, that very different methods will be required. The patient already knows, as well as the prieft and moralift, that the indulgence is pernicious, and ultimately fatal : he is alfo aware, without the reafonings of medicine, that the conftant repetition will deftroy health ; but it is not fo eafy to convince him that you poffefs a charm that can recompence his feelings for the want of a grateful ftimulus, or beftow on his nervous fyftem fenfations equally foothing and agreeable as he has been accuftomed to receive from the bewitching fpirit. *Hic labor, hoc opus eft :* this is the difficulty ; this is the tafk, that is to prove your difcernment, patience, and addrefs. That little has been done hitherto with fuccefs, we may be affured, by very rarely meeting with a reformed drunkard. The habit, carried to a certain length, is a gulph, from *whofe bourne no traveller returns ;* where fame, fortune, hope, health, and life perifh.

Amidft the evils which flow from modern wars, is to be reckoned the vaft confumption

of

of spirituous liquors. The tax on distilled spirits forms so large a part of finance, and fills up so great a chasm in the annual budget of any minister, who may strive more to retain his place than to reform the morals, or check the diseases of his countrymen, that we cease to wonder at its continuance. A few years ago, the crops of grain were so deficient over this island, that the distillation of spirits from malt were prohibited : and thus scarcity, bordering on famine, became a blessing to the human race. But no sooner had fruitful seasons, and the bounty of Providence, covered the earth with plenty, than the first gift of Heaven, abundance of corn, was again, for the sake of taxation, converted into poisonous spirits, by opening the stillories. Might not other taxes be devised that would be equally productive ? and would it not be a virtuous act of the Legislature to abolish the practice for ever ?

In order to treat my subject philosophically, and for the sake of method, I propose dividing it into the following heads, viz.

1st, Definition of Drunkenness.

2d,

2d, The Phænomena, or Symptoms of Drunkenneſs.

3d, In what Manner Vinous Spirit affects the living Body.

4th, The Catalogue of Diſeaſes induced by Drunkenneſs. And,

5th, The Method of correcting the Habit of Drunkenneſs, and of treating the Drunken Paroxyſm.

Into theſe heads I ſhall occaſionally introduce ſuch practical remarks as may ariſe out of the ſubject; but which are too deſultory for methodical arrangement.

CHAP.

CHAP. I.

Difinition of Drunkenneſs.

O! thou inviſible ſpirit of Wine, if thou haſt no name to be known
by, let us call thee —— Devil!

SHAKESPEAR.

IN medical language, I conſider drunkenneſs,
ſtrictly ſpeaking, to be a diſeaſe; produced
by a remote cauſe, and giving birth to actions
and movements in the living body, that diſ-
order the functions of health. This being the
caſe, beſides the value of an accurate definition for the ſake of ſyſtem, it may be of
ſome practical utility to point out the affinity
which the paroxyſm has with other affections.
In affigning the character formerly, I was well
aware of the difficulty of fixing on any ſymp-
tom, or even concourſe of ſymptoms, that
are invariably preſent. For this reaſon *delirium*
ſeemed to be the moſt certain, as it is the
moſt prominent and general. But objections
may yet be made to this; for difference of
age, and varieties of temperament and conſtitution, influence the acceffion and progreſs
of

of wavering intellect during intoxication. Again, although the animal functions are evidently deranged, exhibited by all the shades and gradations of *delirium*, such as imbecility of mind or fatuity, erroneous judgment, imaginary perceptions, false relations, violent emotions called raving, &c. yet at the same time, the paroxysm is so generally attended with a partial or total abolition of the powers of sense and motion, that it assumes very much the nature of a *comatose* condition. Indeed the most frequent fatal termination of the drunken fit is apoplexy. It is certainly no uncommon occurrence to see an inebriate who can neither walk or speak, exercise so considerable a degree of mental power, as to recollect every circumstance that passes ; yet so conscious of his inability to move without staggering, that he cunningly watches the opportunity, when unperceived by his companions, to take his leave. The character of this disease therefore, partakes both of *delirium* and *coma*.

To avoid confusion, I take the *remote cause* into my definition. Drunkenness is the delirium occasioned by fermented liquors. It is

true

true that other narcotics, particularly *opium* and *bang*, produce nearly the fame phœno-mena, and their habitual ufe almoft the fame difeafes ; yet, for obvions reafons, the chief of which is the common occurrence of drunken-nefs in this country, I am induced to feparate them here, and confider this fubject by itfelf. —— Our definition is briefly this :

POST VINUM IMMODICE ASSUMPTUM, DELIRIUM ET COMA.—Which may be thus tranflated :—" Imbecility of intellect, erro-" neous judgment, violent emotions ; and lofs " of fenfe and motion after the immoderate " ufe of vinous liquors."

The Latin word " Vinum," has been pre-ferred as being the moft concife, and beft conveying the meaning of vinous fpirit, the product of fermentation, and on which the inebriating power of all fermented liquors depends ; fuch as wine, malt-liquors, cyder, perry, mum, mead, koumifs, &c. all of which by diftillation yield alkohol.

The *carbonic acid gas, or fixed air*, which is evolved in great quantity during the vinous fermentation, that gives a fparkling and pun-gency to certain liquors, fuch as champaigne,

bottled

bottled beer and cyder, is known to produce a kind of ftupefaction refembling intoxication, independent of the fpirit. This kind of ebriety is but momentary; as the action of the gas on the nerves of the ftomach is of fhort duration. Very different are the effects of this *gas* when breathed. Brewers have frequently been fuffocated in taking out their ale or beer from the vat, as the air lies on the furface of the fermenting liquor. Nay it has fometimes accumulated in fuch quantities in clofe cellars, as to prove fatal to feveral people before the caufe was detected, and the air expelled by ventilation. In mines, wells, and the holds of fhips, this vapour has often proved lethalic.

Dr. Cullen, in his order of *Vefaniæ*, or mental derangement, has given five genera: but the paroxyfm of ebriety more particularly exemplifies the mixed character of *amentia*, *infania et mania*, or ideotifm, agreeable emotions, and violent emotions. *Oneirodynia*, difturbed fleep, which comprehends fleep-walking and night-mare, perhaps only occurs during the decline of the drunken paroxyfm. And *melancholia*, melancholy, would appear

7   to

to be fufpended during the ftimulant power
of wine. This difeafe is rather the offspring
of habitual intoxication ; it is probably confined to a peculiar temperament of body, that
is little difpofed to be excited, and can endure
exceffive ftimulus without proportional action,
as well in the functions of the *fenforium commune*, as in the circulating fyftem.

There is a fpecies of delirium that often
attends the early acceffion of *typhus fever*,
from contagion that I have known to be
miftaken for ebriety. Among feamen and
foldiers, where habits of intoxication are common, it will fometimes require nice difcernment
to decide ; for the vacant ftare in the countenance, the look of ideotifm, incoherent
fpeech, faultering voice, and tottering walk,
are fo alike in both cafes, that the naval and
military furgeon ought at all times to be very
cautious, how he gives up a man to punifhment under thefe fufpicious appearances.
Nay, the certainty of his having come from a
tavern, with even the effluvium of liquor
about him, are figns not always to be trufted :
for thefe haunts of feamen and foldiers are
often the fources of infection. In all doubtful

ful cafes of this kind, let the members of our profeffion be guarded in their opinions; it is fafe to lean to the humane fide.

There is another fpecies of intoxication that follows the inhalation of inflammable fpirit, by the nofe and mouth, without being fwallowed. This fpecies of ebriety is common to coopers, porters, and other workmen employed in cellars and diftilleries. The moft volatile part of the fpirit, or pureft alkohol, which arifes in pouring it from one veffel to another, probably acts by directly ftimulating the nerves of the *membrana Shneideriana* fpread about the nofe and frontal finufes; and alfo the infide of the mouth, trachea and lungs, and thus produces delirium. This ebriety is likewife tranfitory, and foon difappears when the patient is moved into the open air. It frequently happens in fhips, in pumping fpirits from a large cafk into a fmaller, in the confined fpace of a fpirit room: but the practice is dangerous, as veffels have often been fet on fire by a lighted candle touching the fpirits; and it is now ftrictly forbidden in all well regulated fhips in his Majefty's navy.

CHAP.

CHAP. II.

Phænomena and Symptoms of Drunkenneſs.

Huc, Pater O Lenæe, veni: nudataque muſto
Tinge novo mecum correptis crura cothurnis. Virg.

THE firſt effects of wine are, an inexpreſſible tranquillity of mind, and livelineſs of
countenance: the powers of imagination become more vivid, and the flow of ſpirits more
ſpontaneous and eaſy, giving birth to wit and
humour without heſitation. *Diſſipat Evrius
curas edaces.* All anxieties of buſineſs, that
require thought and attention, are laid aſide;
and every painful affection of the ſoul is relieved or alleviated. Placed, as it were, in a
paradiſe of pleaſure, the being only contem-
plates delightful and agreeable objects; the
moſt prominent of them are love and deſire,

———— ſine Baccho friget Venus.

Ter.

The man of a lively fancy, who happens
to be in love at ſuch a time, ſees beauties in
his

his miftrefs that he overlooked before; and he culls every flower of poefy that can add warmth to his emotions, or paffion to his feelings. The delirium of love may, therefore, be faid to begin firft.

An agreeable heat is diffufed over the whole body; mufcular ftrength is recruited, and the action of the heart and arteries is manifeftly increafed.

The vigour of the circulation of the blood, being thus augmented, a fparkling of the eyes may be obferved; a flufh or rednefs is fpread over the face, and the whole appearance of the countenance is brightened into a fmile.

A painter, fuch as Hogarth, would find fine exercife for his talents in delineating the fhades and gradations of feature that take place in particular perfons, from perfect fobriety to the laft ftage of intoxication. The foul, as if unconfcious of its danger, looks with bodily organs that befpeak rapture to the deceitful bowl, which carries in its draught every degree of fenfation, from pleafure to pain, from the pureft perceptions of intellect, to the laft confufion of thought; which raifes man above the fphere of mortals, and

ends

ends, by bringing him to a level with the brutes.

When the mind has attained the higheſt degree of pleaſurable feeling from vinous ſtimulus, it is wrapt in *reverie*, which may be called a boundary, between the agreeable ſenſations of ſobriety, and the delirious tumults of thought, which uſher in complete inebriation. The ſyſtem has been enough excited to bring forth pleaſurable ſenſation, to ſubdue pain, and ſufficient judgment remains to analize the reflections which ariſe from condition of life, ſo as to fortify the preſent moment againſt all the intruſive approaches of care or ſorrow. Did the giddy votaries of Bacchus but ſtop here, ſome indulgence might be granted, that human nature ſhould a while forget thoſe ills which fleſh is heir to.

During this period, which I muſt beg leave to call the *drunken reverie*, that diſguiſe which all mankind, more or leſs, carry about them, is in ſome meaſure thrown off. The grave philoſopher himſelf, becomes convivial, lays aſide his ſevere demeanour, and applauds the jeſt and the ſong.

——Teucer

—— Teucer Salamina patremque
Cum fugerit tamen uda Lyæo
Tempora populea fertur vinxiſſe corona.   Hor.

Narratur et priſci Catonis
Sæpe mero caluiſſe virtus.   Hor.

Invigorated with wine, the infirm man becomes ſtrong, and the timid courageous. The deſponding lover forſakes his ſolitude, and ſilent ſhades, and in a cup of Falernian forgets the frowns and indifference of an unkind miſtreſs. Even the trembling hypochondriac, unmindful of his fears and ominous dreams, ſports and capers like a perſon in health. Regaled with the pleaſures of the board, the ſoldier no longer complains of the hardſhips of a campaign, or the mariner of the dangers of the ſtorm.

Quis poſt vina gravem militiam aut pauperiem crepat ?   Hor.

Vino pellite curas
Cras ingens iterabimus equor.   Hor.

Such appear to be the chearful and inſpiring powers of wine. All beyond ſeem to be chaos and madneſs. " Tria ego pocula
       c   " tantum

" tantum mifceo, illis qui fapiunt; unum fa-
" nitatis ; alterum voluptatis ; foporis tertium,
" &c.* " " Give ftrong drink unto him that
" is ready to perifh; and wine unto thofe
" that be of heavy heart. Let him drink
" and forget his poverty, and remember his
" mifery no more †." So fpake the royal
voluptuary, who planted him vineyards, and
gave himfelf unto wine : yet he foon found,
as every drunkard has done fince, that " all
" was vanity and vexation of fpirit."

A lover of the bottle, a jolly companion as
commonly expreffed, would give you juft fuch
a defcription of the effects of wine, as Shakefpear has put into the mouth of the maudlin
Falftaff. " Good faith, this fame young fo-
" ber-blooded boy doth not love me; nor a
" man cannot make him laugh :—but that's
" no marvel; he drinks no wine. There's
" never any of thefe demure boys come to
" any proof : for thin drink doth fo overcool
" their blood, and making many fifh meals,
" that they fall into a kind of male green-fick-

* Eubul.   † Proverbs.

nefs :

" nefs: and then when they marry, *they get*
" *wenches* : * they are generally fools and
" cowards; which fome of us fhould be too,
" but for inflammation. A good fherries
" fack hath a two-fold operation in it. It
" afcends me into the brain ; dries there all the
" foolifh, and dull, and crudy vapours which
" environ it ; makes it apprehenfive, quick,

---

* " If a drunken man get a child, it will never likely
" have a good brain," as Gellius argues. Lib. xii. cap. 1.
" *Ebrii gignunt ebrios*, one drunkard begets another," faith
Plutarch :—and Ariftotle himfelf admits, that " drunken
" women bring forth children like unto themfelves."
Burton Anat. Mel.

If thefe authorities, along with Sir John Falftaff's, can
have any weight, mankind have a ftronger reafon againft
intoxication, than has ufually been urged by moral writers.
That is the dread of tranfmitting *infanity* to their offspring.
Dr. Darwin, in his reveries about generation, fpeaks of the
progeny receiving likenefs of form from the imagination
of the parent. But if imagination can have the power of
impreffing the *fhapelefs ens*, how much more muft the real
condition of the inebriate. The legiflators of fome countries had fuch ideas of the effects of wine, as being a poifon
to the foul and a fomentor of vices, that their women
were fubjected to the fame punifhment for drinking as for
adultery. Gel. lib. x. cap. 23. Whatever may be the
truth of this doctrine, fobriety in hufband and wife muft
give the beft chance for a fober progeny. Dr. Darwin even
fays, " It is remarkable that all the difeafes from drinking
" fpirituous or fermented liquors are liable to become he-
" reditary, even to the third generation, gradually increaf-
" ing, if the caufe be continued, till the family becomes
" extinct." Bot. Gard. Part ii. Note on *Vitis*.

" forgetive,

" forgetive, full of nimble, fiery, and delect-
" able fhapes; which delivered over to the
" voice (the tongue), which is the birth, be-
" comes excellent wit. The fecond property
" of your excellent fherries is, the warm-
" ing of the blood; which before, cold and
" fettled, left the liver white and pale; which
" is the badge of pufillanimity and cowardice:
" but the fherries warms it, and makes it
" courfe from the inwards to the parts ex-
" treme. It illumineth the face; which, as a
" beacon, gives warning to all the reft of this
" little kingdom man, to arm: and then the
" vital commoners, and inland petty fpirits,
" mufter me all to their captain the heart;
" who great, and puffed up with this retinue,
" doth any deed of courage; and this valour
" comes of fherries: fo that fkill in the wea-
" pon is nothing without fack; for that fets
" it a work; learning a mere hoard of gold
" kept by a devil, till fack commences it and
" fets it in act and ufe. Hereof comes it that
" prince Harry is valiant; for the cold blood
" he did naturally inherit of his father, he
" hath, like lean, fterile, and bare land, ma-
" nured, hufbanded, and tilled, with excellent

4   " endeavour

" endeavour of drinking good, and good ſtore
" of fertile ſherries: that he is become very
" hot and valiant. If I had a thouſand ſons,
" the firſt human principle I would teach
" them, ſhould be,—to forſwear thin potation,
" and to addict themſelves to ſack."

Hen. iv. *part* ii. *act* 4.

The ſober pleaſures of Bacchus have now
been detailed ; noiſy folly and ribaldry next
appear : the ſong becomes louder, and dancing commences with the rude ſqueeze, and
every odd geſticulation ; chearfulneſs and
wit are changed into low humour and ob-
ſcene jeſts.

> ———— tollite barbarum
> Morem, verecundumque Bacchum,
> Sanguineis prohibite rixis. Hor.

The man is now drunk, and whatever he
ſays or does, betrays the errors of the thinking principle. This ſcene is finely painted by
Thomſon in his poem of the Seaſons ; and as
it is far beyond the compaſs of medical or
technical language, I ſhall give it in his own
words :

———But

——— But earnest brimming bowls
Lave every soul, the table floating round,
And pavement faithless to the fuddled foot.
Thus as they swim in mutual swil, the talk,
Vociferous at once from twenty tongues
Reels fast from theme to theme, from horses, hounds,
To church or mistress, politics or ghost,
In endless mazes intricate, perplex'd.
Mean time, with sudden interruption loud,
Th' impatient catch bursts from the joyous heart ;
That moment touch'd is every kindred soul ;
And opening in a full-mouth'd cry of joy,
The laugh, the slap, the jocund curse go round.

Along with this noise and folly, all the weaknesses of disposition are unveiled, and the secrets of the breast are exposed without reserve. He must be a fool indeed, who shall expound to a rival, the *arcana* of his profession, of his love, or of his friendship ! hence the old adage, " *in vino veritas.*"

Condita cum verax operit præcordia Liber.   Hor.

From this circumstance, it is finely recorded of the Roman chief, that he proved the confidence and sincerity of his counsellors by wine, before he ventured to trust them.

Religious enthusiasm is apt to occupy the imagination of fanatics at this time, and they burst burft forth with blafphemous and familiar addreffes to the deity. Their hypocrify has loft its veil; they have now the audacity to talk of vifitations from heaven, and the infpirations of the fpirit, in all the impudent and unintelligible cant of their fect.

The cultivated mind is even feen in drunkennefs. It commits no outrage, provokes no quarrel, and turns its ear from infult and offence. But the ignorant and illiterate man is to be fhunned in proportion to his excefs : it is human nature in its vileft garb, and madnefs in its worft form.

There feems no phyfical ftrength of conftitution that can fufficiently guard againft the expofure of thefe frailties of difpofition; the moft torpid feelings difcover the infirmity. But there is one trait of the moral character, that I have obferved, proof againft them. It is notorious in the gamefter, that he fhuns drinking; but plies his companions with the bottle, that he may fecure fome advantage to himfelf. I fpeak here of gaming as a fpecies of avarice. The avaricious man, when drunk, never tells a fecret of his foul. Avarice is a paffion of fo mean a nature, that it will flou-

rifh

rish where no other can grow; no mental soil
is so steril not to nourish it. A smaller portion of intellect is required for its exercise
than for any other vice. As it is so completely environed by self, it feels for no fel-
low-creature: in all conditions of life it looks
at home: when sober, it displays no charity,
and never needs to repent of profusion. During drunkenness, the ruling passion is steady
to its purpose; " *virtus post nummos:*" it is always prepared to take advantage of a drunken
brother; and whether it fleeces him at
games of chance, or overreaches him by the
tricks of a bargain, you perceive the grasp of
avarice, as true to the lust of gain, amidst the
delirious excesses of the bottle, as the magnet
to the pole, in a storm at sea. " *Qui lædit*
temulentum prodit absentem."

In the heat of intoxication, supposed af-
fronts, that had never been noticed by the
party before, are called up, to claim an apology, or provoke a quarrel. Resentments that
had been long suppressed, or apparently for-
gotten, are brought to recollection, that they
may seek revenge, or meet with redress.
These give birth to numerous feuds and ani-
mosities,

mofities, which frequently terminate in blood-fhed and death.

Some conditions of body alfo mark and accompany this degree of ebriety. As ftupor fupervenes, voluntary motion being partly loft, the head nods, the walk is tottering, *vox faucibus hæret* *. The countenance looks fwoln and inflamed, the eyes ftart and glare, vifion is double †; or is rendered obfcure, from mifts or meteors, flying, as it were, in the atmofphere.

> ———— Their feeble tongues,
> Unable to take up the cumbrous word,
> Lie quite diffolv'd. Before their maudlin eyes,
> Seen dim and blue, the double tapers dance,
> Like the fun wading through the mifty fky.
>
> THOMSON.

Et ebrius interdum improvifo minget, et alvum exonerat. Thefe imbecilities are the confequence of the lofs of power in the fphincter mufcles: they are peculiar to certain perfons. Even voracious appetite, fuch as is fometimes obferved in the apopleclic ftate, is no unfrequent occurrence in this ftage of ebriety.

---

* Aphonia temulentorum. Sauv. f. 3.
† Diplopia a temulentia. Sauv. Var. 10.

Such

Such are the chief phænomena of drunkenness; but they vary confiderably in different perfons, and very much depend on the natural difpofition and temperament. We thus fee fome men, in their cups, mild, good-natured, and gentle; while others are fierce, irrafcible, and implacable: this one is complaifant to his enemy, and forgetful of injuries; that, is infulting to his friend, and mindful of revenge. This perfon is gay, mufical, and loquacious; that one is dull, fullen, and filent. Here, a drunkard weeps and moans with wry faces; there, another turbulent and loud, foaming with rage, makes the dome echo with oaths and imprecations. As in every other fpecies of infanity, fo in thefe moments the inebriate forgets the blufh of ingenuous fhame, and commits many indecent actions.

How dreadful the lot of that man, who, while heated and mad with wine, fhall plunge his fword into the bofom of his friend! In fuch an hour the infuriate Alexander flew his moft dear companion Clytus!

The doctrine of temperaments is not well underftood: and it would be difficult to explain

plain the peculiar actions of persons during
the influence of wine, by the induction of this
doctrine. The sanguineous and choleric temperaments, I conceive to be most prone to re-
sentment and ferocity; as may be observed in
those whose countenance becomes very much
flushed or bloated, with their eyes as if start-
ing from their sockets : the former of the two
is the most lascivious and amorous. The
nervous temperament exhibits most signs of
idiotism, and is childish and foolish in its
drunken pranks. The phlegmatic temperament is difficult to be roused ; is passive and
silent, and may fall from the chair before
many external signs of ebriety appear. The
melancholic temperament, as when sober, is
tenacious of whatever it undertakes; and
shews least of the inebriate in its manner.
But all constitutions have something peculiar
to them, and the shades of character blend so
insensibly with one another, that distinction
becomes difficult.

When matters are come to this pass, the
stomach, from being too much overloaded, or
from that debility which follows all excessive
stimulation, is affected with nausea and vomiting.

miting. Should this not happen, sleep quickly seizes the inebriate, and very frequently attended with sterterous breathing. After the space of a few hours, or sooner or later, his senses being recovered, but without recollection of what has passed, the drunkard awakes, languid, low-spirited, and much debilitated.

Here the paroxysm may be said to terminate, and more or less of febrile affection commences: from whence are produced, sensibility to the external air, chills, shivering, creeping on the skin, weakness, inactivity of body and mind, heaviness and pain of the head, nausea, thirst, vomiting, small pulse, for the most part frequent, with many other signs of debility.

The drunken paroxysm, as far as can be observed in those who are addicted to the habit, has some variation from the history now given of the phænomena. The chearfulness of mind, and lively countenance, with all the agreeable and pleasurable feelings, are by no means exhibited in the same degree. In short, like all human enjoyments, the exhilarating powers of wine lose their fine zest

and

and high relifh, by being too frequently indulged. This very circumftance at once draws
the line between the temperate man and the
fot.

It ought to be remembered, that the fame
quantity of wine, or vinous fpirit, will not
always produce the fame effects in the fame
perfons; or in the fame man at all times.
This muft depend on the habit of intoxication; the ftomach being full or empty; the
ufual hour of drinking; a cold or warm
country; the temperature of the room; the
fummer or winter feafon; fafting, or after a
repaft; and finally, by whatever means the
ftate of the body increafes or diminifhes
the action of ftimuli. This is the fcale of
excitability, as explained by Brown in his
Elementa Medicinæ.

The moft fotted drunkard knows well that
a fmaller quantity of fpirit will do his bufinefs
in a morning than after he has dined. Hence
a rule in temperance never to drink wine on
an empty ftomach; or after very long fafting.
A very ftriking fact to this purpofe, is to be
found in Captain Bligh's narrative of his paffage to Timor, after the mutiny on board the
Bounty.

Bounty. The allowance of water and provision was so exceedingly small, that it was little better than fasting. The rum was measured by a tea spoon; yet the body was so susceptible of stimulus, that this quantity produced inebriation. This condition has been called accumulated excitability.

Again, persons labouring under typhus fever very frequently consume from four to six pounds of wine in the twenty-four hours; not only without stupor supervening, but delirium, such as it is in that disease, disappearing; and the frequency of the pulse diminishing in proportion at the same time. The use of wine as a cordial in fever is of very ancient date. Pliny the elder says:— " Cardiacorum morbo, unicam spem in vino " esse, certum est [*]." Aretaus, and Cælius Aurelianus give similar evidence. In my own practice, supported by experience more extensive than that of any physician of the present age, it has been my chief remedy; and when directed with due precaution, by far the most efficacious in the low typhus fever [†].

[*] Plin. Nat. Hist. lib. xxiii. c. 2.
[†] Vide Medicina Nautica, vol. i. art. *Typhus*.

CHAP.

CHAP. III.

In what Manner vinous Spirit affects the Body.

Every inordinate cup is unbleſſed, and the ingredient is a—devil!
SHAKESPEAR.

IN the preceding chapter I have detailed the effects of wine in the living human body, as far as feemed neceffary for marking the phænomena which take place from perfect fobriety, to the ftate of intoxication and total infenfibility.

The firft effect to be perceived is ftimulant and exciting; calling forth vigour of body and mind, pleafurable fenfation, and power of intellect. The next is lofs of voluntary motion, and delirium. The laft is a ftate of indirect debility, or exhaufted excitability, from inordinate action of the different functions.

The inebriating quality of all liquors, I have faid, depends upon the ALKOHOL which they contain. This word is of Arabic origin;
for

for the Arabians firſt obtained alkohol from wine. It means the *pure ſpirit* ſeparated by repeated diſtillations from all groſſer matter. It is the product of the vinous fermentation from ſugar, and can only be obtained from thoſe ſubſtances which poſſeſs the ſaccharine principle.

As an article in *materia medica*, phyſicians have referred alkohol to the claſs of *narcotics ;* medicines which induce ſtupor and ſleep, among which are reckoned opium, bangue, cicuta, belladonna, hyoſciamus, nicotiana, lauroceraſus, &c.

The operation of *narcotics* has lately given birth to much controverſy in medical writings; the one party contending for a *primary ſedative* power in theſe medicines, which by ſuſpending ſenſe and motion, that condition of the body takes place which is called *ſleep.* On the other hand it is argued, that the firſt effects of *narcotics* are ſtimulant and exciting ; and that *ſleep* only comes on as a conſequence of preceding excitement: they are therefore to be conſidered as only *indirectly ſedatives.* Experiments have been inſtituted by both parties, from which each have drawn concluſions

favourable

favourable to their own fide of the queftion.
In difputes of this nature, preconceived theories, attachment to particular doctrines, and
favourite modes of reafoning, have had great
influence in prejudicing the minds of the different combatants, and thus giving birth to
feeming contradictions. But there is one
point in which they nearly agree, and which
feems fufficient for the purpofe of the practical phyfician. It is admitted, I think on all
hands, that narcotic medicines, or I will take
the chief of them, opium, is univerfally found
to be hurtful and improper, in all *fthenic* difeafes, or thofe reputed to be inflammatory in
their nature. Who ever thinks of prefcribing
opium in pneumonia? in phrenitis, or in
acute rheumatifm previous to venæfection and
other evacuations? What reafons are affigned
for this caution? They are obvious: In
pneumonia, opium increafes the difficulty of
expectoration and breathing, and anxiety; in
phrenitis it exalts the delirium and reftleff-
nefs; and in acute rheumatifm, the fever,
pain, and heat of the body, become more
fevere after its exhibition. Thefe effects are

D   produced

produced by a general ftimulant power, fpread
over the whole body, but particularly exemplified in the circulating fyftem. The ftroke
of the artery becomes either fuller or more
oppreffed; the lungs are overloaded with
blood, and incapable of due expanfion; the
blood is alfo accumulated in the head, apparent from the flufh of the countenance and
rednefs of the eyes, and throbbing of the
temporal arteries; the circulation being alfo
increafed in the joints, gives additional heat
and pain. The phyfician who thus decides
from fick-bed experience, wifely withholds
opium in all fuch conditions of body.

But in another ftate of the body, very oppofite to the difeafes juft mentioned; and
often independent of all authorities of phyficians, various fubftances of this clafs are ufed
by the inhabitants of different countries, as
opium and bang by the Turks and Eaft Indians, and tobacco by all others. Thefe articles are certainly not taken in this manner,
either for their antifpafmodic or fedative virtues : but as ftimulants and cordials, that give
vigour to the fyftem, raife the fpirits, call
forth

forth agreeable feelings, and render the body, for a time, capable to bear fatigue and privation of food.

Opium, it is well known, is the juice obtained from the feed-pod of the white poppy, papaver fomniferum Lin. S. P. and when taken in due quantity is very analogous in its action to ardent fpirit. Bang, or bangue, is made from the leaf of a wild kind of hemp, that grows in the countries of the Levant. It is firft dried and then pulverized. The effects of this drug are to confound the underftanding ; fet the imagination loofe ; induce a kind of folly and forgetfulnefs, wherein all cares are left, and joy and gaiety take place thereof. Bang in reality is a fuccedaneum to wine, and obtains in thofe countries where mahometanifm is eftablifhed; which prohibiting the ufe of that liquor abfolutely, the poor Muffulmans are forced to have recourfe to fuccedanea to roufe their fpirits *.

In a large dofe thefe fubftances bring on delirium, ftupor, and other phænomena of ebriety. Their habitual ufe caufes uni-

* Ency. Brit.

verfal

verfal debility, emaciation, lofs of intellect, palfy, dropfy, dyfpepfia, hepatic difeafes, and all others which flow from indulgence of fpirituous liquors. I may therefore conclude, that all narcotics have more or lefs the fame effect.

From thefe articles, and fome others of the fame clafs, alkohol chiefly differs, by being taken generally in a diluted ftate, fuch as in wine, beer, or punch, and ufed as an ingredient in diet. Highly rectified fpirit, or pure alkohol, could fcarcely be admitted into the human ftomach, even in very moderate quantity, without proving immediately fatal. The coats of the ftomach would be unable to refift fo concentrated a ftimulus; they would be inftantly decompounded, as is done by nitric or fulphuric acids. When given by drops like tinct. opii, in any convenient drink, this pure alkohol will prove equally ferviceable in allaying pain, in increafing the ftrength and velocity of the pulfe, raifing the fpirits, &c. and would be called antifpafmodic. But to fhow how inconclufive much of the reafoning is, which has been employed here; the fupporters of the fedative doctrine, do do not deny a directly ftimulant power to all vinous liquors. The effects of opium, I confider nearly alike to thofe of ardent fpirit. The opium eaters among the Turks, give evidence of this fubftance increafing defire, and the fexual appetite, like wine in moderate quantities ; but deftroying the paffion when long ufed, or too largely employed. It is well known that many of our fair countrywomen carry laudanum about with them, and take it freely when under low fpirits. This cuftom is certainly as little to be juftified as the ufe of brandy. Were opium a fedative, how could it poffefs thofe powers, evidently ftimulating to the bodies of perfons who never troubled themfelves about the difputes concerning the mode of action, and who could be biaffed by no theoretical opinion.

There are fome liquors which have a hurtful tendency, independent of the fpirituous quality. The malt liquors, and cyder of this country, do not undergo fo perfect a fermentation, as the product of the grape in warmer latitudes. The firft is therefore apt to diforder the ftomach, by a flight fermentation afterwards in the body: this is a procefs that

perfons

persons of weak degestive organs cannot suffer
without much pain. The carbonic acid gas
which is there disengaged, excites gastrodynia,
flatulency, and distension; but we are acquainted with no virtues which this gas possesses beyond a slight stimulus; the modern
practice of exhibiting it so often, and in various ways, has rather arisen from the rage after
chemical remedies, than any fair evidence that
has been given of its medical qualities. The
cyders of England, and America, and I rather
suppose of all countries, are impregnated with
much undecompounded acid: the apple yields
but a small quantity of saccharine matter, at
least not sufficient by its fermentative quality
to overcome the whole of the malic acid
which abounds in the fruit, and thus convert
it into vinous spirit. But beer, and particularly porter, have their narcotic power much
increased by noxious compounds which enter
them; and the bitters which are necessary to
their preservation, by long use, injure the
nerves of the stomach, and add to the stu-
pefactive quality. Malt-liquor drinkers are
known to be prone to apoplexy and palsy,
from this very cause: and purl drinkers in a

still

ftill greater degree, a mixture peculiar to this country. This poifonous morning beverage was, till lately, confined to the metropolis and its vicinity; but has now, like other luxuries, found its way into all provincial towns.

The legiflature has lately turned its attention to the noxious quality of fome of the porter brewed in London; and opium has been mentioned as an ingredient frequently added to this liquor. An increafe of duty has been laid on this celebrated drug by way of prohibition. But when we confider that four grains of opium are fufficient, to double the intoxicating power of a gallon of porter, the article is ftill cheap enough to be ufed by the brewer, without fubtracting much of his profits. The increafed duty will alfo increafe the temptation to fmuggle. The Minifter of the prefent day is a profeffed phyfician, and once prefcribed a *hop pillow* to an *illuftrious patient*. May Heaven direct, that the Hopes with which he now pillows that facred head, may not turn out a *bitter pillow!* But Mr. Addington does not feem to have been aware, that while he was taking opium from the

D 4 brewers,

brewers, he left them in full poffeffion of a long lift of narcotics. They have the *Coculus Indicus*, dog-poifon, which is faid to be their favourite ingredient: they have alfo hyofci-amus, belladowna, and lauro-cerafus; all of which are cheap; and could they not alfo pro-cure, at a low price, bangue from the Levant, which many Mahometans prefer to opium it-felf? I believe bitters of all kinds, long con-tinued, are hurtful to the nervous fyftem; it is difficult to fay which of them ought to be preferred as being moft falutary. Hop is cer-tainly one of the moft grateful, but poffeffes no fuperior efficacy as an antizymic. It is an article on which Government can levy a duty with more certainty than on any other, and its bulk and mode of growth preclude fmuggling; but thefe feem the chief reafons for the preference. Again, while the Minifter was commendably employed in checking the nefarious traffic of the brewers, he forgot that he was wrefting from the bed of pain and ficknefs, by increafing its price, an article that is the laft refuge of our art; that fortifies the foul againft the pangs of feparation from the

body,

body, and as it were prunes its wings for its flight to another world! But, to return to my fubject:

The operation of vinous fpirit on the body is twofold; which may be divided into

I. Intoxicating; and,
II. Chemical.

Intoxication or drunkennefs is the delirium which fucceeds the immediate ufe of fermented liquors or wine. It is " *delirium ferox;*" it is the ferocious delirium of authors, to diftinguifh it from the mild delirium, " *delirium mite,*" fuch as attends the fever from typhoid contagion.

It would be an endlefs digreffion, and very little ufeful to the prefent inveftigation, to detail the various theories and conjectures of phyficians and metaphyficians on the connection between body and mind. That our intellectual part can be difturbed, and fo completely deranged, by bodily difeafes, as to be incapable of ufing its reafoning powers, is a fact fufficiently eftablifhed to be univerfally admitted. But to offer opinions on the nature of a foul, of a nervous power, or of a fentient principle,

principle, is not the intention of this work. I
shall therefore confine myself to the humbler,
but more useful task, of gleaning the field of
inquiry for scattered facts, and endeavour to
collect them into a groupe.

The stimulant action of ardent spirit is first
exerted on the stomach, and spread, by sym-
pathy, from thence to the *sensorium commune*,
and the rest of the system. But there can be
no doubt that much of the liquor also enters
the circulation, and gives there an additional
stimulus : for we are acquainted with no particular appetency inherent in the lacteal vessels, that can confine the absorption only to
mild and bland fluids. It is true that the
urine, perspirable matter, and serum of inebriates, have never yet been so carefully ana-
lized as to discover alkohol ; but that vinous
spirit mixes with the blood we know to a
certainty, from the hydrogenous gas which
escapes from the lungs, to be perceived in the
fœtor of the breath. We are, however, ignorant what combinations the hydrogene, or
other parts of the alkohol, may form with the
human fluids. But, besides the effect which
spirits may have, in directly exciting the ner-

vous fyftem, it would appear that intoxication and delirium are alfo much increafed, by the force of the circulation in the blood veffels of the brain, and the mechanical compreffion as a confequence of their furcharged ftate. This being admitted, at once explains why fo much comatofe affection attends ebriety. It is alfo obferved that fome liquors, more than others, produce fopor: porter, and all ftrong malt liquors, are of this defcription, as characterifed by the fwoln and bloated countenance, ftupor, fluggifhnefs, drowfinefs, and fleep: while gaiety and an immenfe flow of fpirits diftinguifh the frifhy delirium from drinking champaigne, and fome other liquors. Obefity and fullnefs commonly follow the long indulgence of ftrong ale, ftrong beer, or porter: the blood veffels would appear to be clogged with a denfe blood; and I have obferved, in fuch cafes, that the drunken paroxyfm lafts much longer, than when it has been produced by any kind of wine, or even ardent fpirit diluted or otherwife. The fixed air in champaigne muft give but a temporary ftimulus; and the tartar, which is an ingredient in all wines,

probably

probably facilitates their evacuation from the body, by its diuretic quality.

Indeed the only way of accounting for the folution of the drunken paroxyfm, muft be as follows : the ardent fpirit muft either be attenuated, diluted, neutralized, or evacuated, that it ceafes to have effect. It probably partakes of all thefe. It is alfo peculiar to the living fibre, to remain a given time in the ftate of excitement only, unlefs a new portion of ftimulus is fupplied. But the body does not immediately return to the former condition after the folution of the difeafe. It has been weakened by exceffive ftimulation ; and it is only by the exhibition of moderate ftimuli, fuch as pure air, animal food, and mental exhilaration, that it can refume its former health and vigour. The head-ach, naufea, languor, and low-fpirits, which follow a debauch, are fo many proofs of a debilitated frame. The fot is then a fubject for the prefcription of Horace :

Toftis marcentem fquillis recreabis, et Afra
Potorem cochleâ : nam lactuca innatat acri
Poft vinum ftomacho: perna magis, ac magis hillis
Flagitat immorfus refici : ——

The

The difciples of the late Dr. Brown, author of *Elementa Medicinæ*, fome of thefe, men of great genius and learning, were always at a lofs to explain the fcale of exciting power on the excitability, by demonftration. Thus, if you begin at good health, and ftimulate a man up to any fthenic difeafe; afterwards he muft fall to a point beneath what he originally was; and in defcending the fcale he muft at one period of his defcent touch at good health. Now this feems a paradox. The yellow fever is a fthenic difeafe in the firft ftage; in the fecond it is a mixture of fthenic and afthenic; and in the laft it is truly afthenic. Now in its defcent from one end of the fcale to the other, the patient at one time muft have been at the point of good health. Mr. Chriftie, who, I believe, firft contrived to demonftrate this doctrine by a mathematical fcale, fhould have formed it in a circle, which would have exactly anfwered his purpofe. The fit of intoxication is fomewhat analogous to the above defcription of yellow fever.

While the body is under the influence of intoxication, it is furprizing how it will refift impreffions, that at other times would be fatal.

tal. This is particularly the case with respect to contagion, and cold; and perhaps also its infensibility to pain. Men in this condition have certainly, on many occasions, been exposed to typhous contagion, and escaped; while others have suffered: but whether under the same circumstances they would have refifted variolous infection I cannot determine. This being the case, a practice has been inculcated by some physicians, to swallow a little brandy when they approach the sick bed, by way of precaution. With respect to the preference to be given to this mode of prevention, I am not enabled to subscribe, as I have never practised it; but it appears to me rather the placebo of a timid attendant. It is well known that a vigorous circulation of the blood, with that resolution and temper of mind which accompany it, is highly favourable to the resistance of contagion; and such a condition of body and mind may be induced by ardent spirit. But this kind of practice does not agree with my ideas on the subject. A physician in the act of visiting a patient under an infectious disease, whether in an hospital ward, or in a private apartment, ought to consider what
effect

effect his example may have on thofe about him; for whatever he does will be imitated. The ufe of fpirituous liquors, I think, might have bad effects among nurfes and other attendants of the fick. I would much rather inculcate thofe precepts of fecurity, from ventilation and cleanlinefs, &c. which have effected wonders in our naval fervice. I am alfo partial to mental ftimuli, which naturally fpring from the defire of doing our duty. But if at any time thefe fpirits fhould be too freely taken, the debility that fucceeds will more certainly predifpofe the body for the reception of contagion. Perfons under fuch circumftances fhould carefully avoid all communication with infected people, furniture, or cloathing.

The drunkard is alfo found, in the firft ftage of the paroxyfm, to refift the operation of cold. No ftronger proofs of this need be adduced than what are daily obferved among our feamen in the naval fea-ports. Thefe men are permitted to come on fhore to recreate themfelves; but, from a thoughtleffnefs of difpofition, and the cunning addrefs of their landlords, they drink till the laft fhilling

is

is spent; they are then thrust out of the door, and left to pass the night on the pavement. It is surprising how they should escape death on such occasions; for I have known many of them who have slept on the street the greatest part of the night in the severest weather. Nothing but that hardiness of constitution peculiar to the British seamen, which braves every danger, could survive such extremes of cold. During my residence at Plymouth Dock, towards the conclusion of the late war, I had the satisfaction of getting 200 gin-shops shut up. They were destroying the very vitals of our naval service. In the year 1800, not less than one million four hundred thousand pounds prize-money were paid at that port to the seamen; and every trick was practised to entrap those credulous and unthinking people. An overgrown brewer, who had monopolised a number of these houses, complained heavily of my representations to the Admiralty; and said that he had lost 5,000*l.* by the business. It was a most fortunate measure, that such nuisances were corrected before the ships were paid off at the peace.

The

The following fact is a strong instance of the inebriate resisting cold. A miller, very much intoxicated, returning from market late at night, while it snowed and froze hard, missed his way, and fell down a steep bank into the mill-dam. By the fright and sudden immersion, he became so far sensible as to recollect where he was. He then thought the surest way home would be to follow the stream, which would take him within pistol-shot of his own door. Instead, however, of taking that course he waded against the current, without knowing it, till his passage was opposed by a wooden bridge. This bridge he knew; and though he felt some disappointment, he still thought his best way was to follow the stream, for the banks were steep and difficult to climb. He now found himself in a comfortable glow; turned about, and arrived at his own house at midnight, perfectly sober, after having been nearly two hours in the water, and often up to the breech. He went immediately to bed, and rose in perfect health. —As the senses were recovered at the time he got home, it is probable he could not have resisted the cold much longer. This instance

E   tends

tends to confirm a common obfervation, that fudden immerfion in cold water puts a fpeedy end to intoxication.

In an uncommonly cold day, and when fnow and fleet were falling, I found a feaman afleep on the road, moft ftupidly drunk. Afraid that he would foon perifh, I ran to the guard-houfe, and procured two foldiers to carry him into a houfe. We fucceeded in getting him upright; but the moment he faw foldiers about him, the dread of becoming their pri-foner fo far operated, that he recovered the ufe of his limbs, and fled from them with the utmoft fpeed, and did not ftop till he thought himfelf out of their reach. I came up, and found him again afleep by the fide of a wall. When I roufed him he knew me, and hu-mouroufly remarked, that he had a right to fleep where he pleafed, for he came on fhore *on liberty!*

Infenfibility to pain, in the inebriated ftate, is daily exemplified, by the moft dreadful bruifes and wounds being inflicted without the fmalleft figns of feeling, and generally without recollection. Cafes of this kind are more frequent among feamen than any where elfe:

elſe: their heedleſs revels expoſe them to more diſaſters than other deſcriptions of mankind. A fatal wound is thus often received without the ſlighteſt recollection how it was done.

A ſailor belonging to a king's ſhip, in which I then ſerved, while drunk, quarrelled with his wife; and, in the fury of paſſion, ſeized a butcher's cleaver, and cut off two of his fingers by the root. The wounds were dreſſed and the man put to bed. When he waked in the morning, he had no remembrance of what happened; ſhowed the utmoſt contrition, and wept like a child for his misfortune when he was told that he had done it himſelf.

Many curious anecdotes might be collected of drunken people, that could not we'l be arranged among the uſual phænomena. Men of uncultivated minds exhibit moſt ſigns of outrage and ferocity; and are certainly the moſt dangerous. Drunkenneſs has been called a vice of barbarous and uncivilized nations *; for ſavages in the ſtate of intoxica-

* Robertſon's America, book iv. Forſter's Voyage, page 481.

tion

tion are like fo many devils. But Chriftians have little reafon to charge the Negro and Indian with the propenfity to intoxication, while it prevails fo much among themfelves. I have known a drunken man whip a poft till he was tired, which he took for a human being that would not move out of his way. An old gentleman of 80, when in his cups, became fo amorous, as to take a lamp-poft for a lady, and addreffed it with all the language of paffion and flattery. Dreams are fome-times known to make a ftrong impreffion on the minds of fome people, and it requires a confiderable time to weigh circumftances and compare facts, before they are undeceived. An officer much accuftomed to hard drinking, after getting intoxicated at the mefs-table, fell afleep; and awoke fuddenly at the end of two hours. He then told one of his brother offi-cers in a peremptory tone of voice, that as it was an affair of honour, now was the beft time for fettling it; and infifted upon their taking their ground immediately. It was with great difficulty that he could be pacified: and no fmall remonftrance took place before he was convinced that he had been dreaming.

The

The following hiſtory of a drunken party
is taken from Burton's Anatomy of Melancholy; a work that abounds with odd ſay-
ings *. " A company of young men at Agri-
" gentum in Sicily came into a tavern ; when,
" after they had freely taken their liquor,
" whether it were the wine itſelf, or ſome-
" thing mixed with it, 'tis not yet known ;
" but upon a ſudden they began to be ſo
" troubled in their brains, that their phanta-
" ſies ſo crazed, that they thought they were
" in a ſhip at ſea ; and now ready to be caſt
" away by reaſon of a tempeſt. Wherefore,
" to avoid ſhipwreck, and prevent drowning,
" they flung all the goods in the houſe out at
" the windows into the ſtreet, or into the ſea,
" as they ſuppoſed : thus they continued mad
" a pretty ſeaſon ; and being brought before
" the magiſtrate to give an account of this
" their faƈt, they told him (not yet reco-
" vered of their madneſs), that what was done
" they did for fear of death, and to avoid
" imminent danger. The ſpeƈtators were all
" amazed at this their ſtupidity ; and gazed
" on them ſtill, whilſt one of the ancienteſt

* Part i. Seƈt. 2. Mem. 5. Subſ. 1.

" of

" of the company, in a grave tone excufed
" himfelf to the magiftrate upon his knees,
" *O ! viri Tritones, ego in imo jacui* ; I befeech
" your Deities, &c. for I was in the bottom
" of the fhip all the while. Another befought
" them as fo many fea-gods, to be good unto
" them ; and if ever he and his fellows came
" to land again, he would build an altar to
" their fervice. The magiftrate could not
" fufficiently laugh at this their madnefs ; bid
" them fleep it out, and went his ways."

This drunken adventure, I believe, was originally told by Plato. The houfe where it
happened was one of the firft in the city ; and
was ever afterwards called *Triremes,* or the
fhip. Brydone, in his *Tour through Sicily,*
gives us an account of another drunken party,
for whom he made punch after the Englifh
form He fays, " We were obliged to re-
" plenifh the bowl fo often, that I really ex-
" pected to fee many of them under the table.
" They called it Pontio (alluding to Pontius
" Pilate), and fpoke loudly in its praife ; de-
" claring that Pontio was a much better fellow
" than they had ever taken him for. How-
" ever, after dinner, one of them, a reverend
" canon,

" canon, grew exceffively fick, and while he
" was throwing up, he turned to me with a
" rueful countenance, and, fhaking his head,
" he groaned out, ' Ah Signor Capitano, fa-
" peva fempre, che Pontio era un grande tra-
" ditore.' ' I always knew that Pontius was
" a great traitor.'—Another, overhearing him,
" exclaimed, ' Afpettativi Signor canonico.'
" Not fo faft, my good canon.' ' Niente al
" pregiudizio di Signor Pontio vi prego.'—
" Recordate che Pontio v' ha fatto un cano-
" nico; et Pontio ha fatto fua excellenza uno
" vefcovo; non fcordatevi mai di voftri ami-
" cis."—*Let.* xx.

From thefe accounts, we muft conclude the
Sicilians are rather a frifky people in their
drunken revels. We thus obferve that the
character of nations, as well as individuals,
may be difcovered in thefe moments. The
defcription which Tacitus gives of a German
caroufal differs confiderably from that of thefe
volatile iflanders; for, according to what he
afferts, deliberations of the moft ferious kind
feem to have been entered upon during ebriety, as well as quarrels and bloodfhed. He
fays, " Diem noctemque, continuare potando,

E 4   " nulli

" nulli probrum.   Crebræ ut inter vinolentos
" rixæ, raro convitiis, fæpius cæde et vulneri-
" bus, tranfiguntur.   Sed et de reconciliandis
" invicem inimicis, et jungendis affinitatibus,
" et adfcifcendis principibus, de pace denique
" ac bello plerumque in conviviis conful-
" tant: tamque nullo magis tempore aut ad
" fimplices cogitationes pateat animus, aut ad
" magnes incalefcat.   Gens non aftuta nec
" callida, aperit adhuc fecreta pectoris licentia
" loci.   Erga detecta et nuda omnium mens,
" poftera die retrahatur: et falva utriufque
" temporis ratio eft.   Deliberant dum fingere
" nefciunt; conftituunt dum errare non pof-
" funt *."   We thus perceive that the frifky
Sicilian, and the fedate German exhibit very
oppofite traits of character, when under the
influence of wine.   Difference of climate, religion, political inftitutions, and cuftoms may
account for this contraft in the difpofition and
paffions of thefe nations ; but fuch an inquiry
is not confiftent with the nature of our work;
it is fufficient to notice the fact.

II. That *alkohol*, independent of its intoxicating quality, poffeffes a *chemical* operation

* Tacitus De Moribus Germanorum.

in

in the human body, cannot be doubted. Applied directly to the animal folid, it conftringes and hardens it; and fufpends its progrefs towards putrefaction when feparated from the body. It coagulates the ferum of the blood, and moft of the fecreted fluids.

Alkohol certainly, deoxygenates the blood in fome degree; at leaft decompounds its floridity. The arterial blood of a profeffed drunkard, approaches to the colour of venous; it is darker than ufual. The rofy colour of the eruptions about the nofe and cheeks does not difprove this: for it is probable that thefe fpots attract oxygen from the atmofphere through the cuticle that covers them, juft as Dr. Prieftly obferved venous blood, confined in a bladder, to acquire a more florid colour from the expofure to his dephlogifticated air *. In the fea fcurvy, a difeafe, where, in the advanced ftage, the blood is always found of a very dark colour, we know that fpirituous liquors more than any thing elfe, have a manifeft tendency to aggravate every fymptom This fact has often come under my obfervation; and a very correct ftatement of

* Prieftley, Experiments on Air.

the

the kind is to be found in my firſt volume on
the Diſeaſes of the Fleet, page 410.

The component parts of alkohol are not
ſufficiently known; but it has a large proportion of hydrogen, which is proved by its
combuſtion in pure air, when water is produced. Thus fourteen ounces of alkohol
burnt in a proper apparatus, with a ſufficient
quantity of oxygen gas, yield ſixteen ounces
of pure water; hydrogen and oxygen being
the component principles of water, as proved
by modern chemiſtry. Alkohol has a ſtrong
attraction for water, and readily mixes with
it, and it is the chief vehicle in which it is
drank; but in what manner it is ſeparated
from the water within the body, would be
difficult to find out. The evolution of hydrogenous gas is chiefly learned from the fœtor
of the breath; it ſeems to be ſent off from
the ſurface of the lungs, in a diſengaged ſtate;
and is often ſo pure in its kind from the ex-
piration of a dram-drinker, that it is eaſily
inflamed on the approach of a candle. The
proceſs of reſpiration probably effects this;
and I ſhould think at ſuch a time there muſt
be an unuſual conſumption of vital air. No
expe-

experiments have been made on the blood of inebriates : and we are not informed, that in the circulating ftate, it exceeds the common temperature of the human body. But it is faid, on the authority of Mr. Spalding the celebrated diver, that after drinking fpirits he always found the air in his bell confumed in a fhorter time, than when he drank water. This gentleman was loft in Dublin bay in 1783, in attempting to take the treafure out of an imperial Indiaman that funk there, on her paffage from Liverpool where fhe was built : the misfortune, it appeared, was owing to the negligence of the attendants in not renewing the air.

If the blood of drunkards is ftrongly charged with hydrogen, muft not that very much affect the quality of the biliary fecretion, independent of any effect it may have on the liver itfelf? Might not the refinous matter which bile is found to contain, be greatly increafed after fpirituous potation? The liver is an organ very liable to be injured by hard drinking; this gives caufe for fufpicion, that the *chemical* operation of alkohol

on

on the blood and the bile, has also some share in producing hepatic diseases. It may increase the generation of *biliary calculi*, and the disposition to dyspepsia, which prevail in the constitution of drunkards.

Is the perspirable matter of drunkards, at all impregnated with hydrogenous gas ?

I am much of opinion that the *chemical* operation of alkohol, has a great influence in retarding the healing of wounds, and in converting them into ulcers. I believe all surgeons agree, that such an effect takes place after hard-drinking, though it is generally attributed to the fever and inflammation which it occasions. The common appearance of eruptions on the surface of the body, may in a great measure be referred to the same source. The exhalations of hydrogenous gas, which arise in some places, are very apt to irritate the eyes, and bring on a painful ophthalmia ; from which it is fair to infer, that the same effect may take place, from blood loaded with hydrogen, circulating through the minute vessels of the *tunica adnata*, as the disease is a common one with wine-bibbers.

The

The fœtor of ulcers, in all drunken subjects, is unusually great; and I shall speak of this under the diseases.

But the most interesting part of this doctrine, is the *combustion of the human body*, produced by the long and immoderate use of spirituous liquors. Such cases are on record; and a collection of them, with remarks, is to be found in the *Journal de Physic*, year 8, by Pierre Aime Lair. I subjoin a copy of that memoir, taken from the Philosophical Magazine, vol. vi. p. 132. by Mr. Alexander Tilloch. It is in vain to request implicit faith to this narrative. The testimony on which the whole cases are given, seems nearly alike. But in the present state of chemistry, and what we know of the nature of spirituous liquors, it does not appear beyond credibility, that from their long and excessive use, such a quantity of hydrogen might accumulate in the body, as to sustain the combustion of it.

It is remarked by some historians when speaking of the death of Alexander the Great, that even in the warm climate of Babylon, his body kept for several days without corruption, from which it has been inferred, that he

did

did not die of poifon, but of hard-drinking *.
That a dead body can be preferved in fpirits of
wine, is well known ; but it is not equally
certain that the body can be preferved by
drinking them before death. It might, however, be a part of the procefs which has been
juft mentioned; the body might be fo far
charged with hydrogen, as to undergo a
flighter combuftion, that might in a manner
toaft it without burning. It is notorious of
this military tiger, that he was a monftrous
drunkard ; and as fond of wine as he was of
human blood. It is to be regretted that his
body could not be preferved to the prefent
day, as it would have filled a niche in the
Louvre for the Firft Conful of France.

Some of my readers may have made the
remark, that the face of particular drunkards, at certain times, appears as much like
a burning coal as any thing can well be conceived. It was probably a face of this kind,
that fuggefted Shakefpear's defcription of Bardolph's nofe. " Falftaff. Thou art our Ad-
" miral, thou beareft the lanthern in the poop,
" but 'tis in the nofe of thee ; thou art the

---

* Robertfon's Hiftory of Greece, p. 427.

" knight

" knight of the burning lamp. I never fee
" thy face but I think upon hell-fire : but for
" the light in thy face, thou art the fon of
" utter darknefs. When thou ran'ft up Gadf-
" hill in the night to catch my horfe, if I did
" not think thou hadft been an *ignis fatuus*,
" or a ball of wild-fire, there's no purchafe
" in money. Thou haft faved me a hundred
" marks in links and torches, walking with
" thee in the night betwixt tavern and tavern :
" but the fack that thou haft drank me, would
" have bought me lights as good cheap, at the
" deareft chandler's in Europe. I have main-
" tained that falamander of your's with fire,
" any time this two-and-thirty years *."

*On the Combuftion of the Human Body, produced
by the long immoderate Ufe of Spirituous Liquors, by* PIERRE AIME LAIR †.

" IN natural as well as civil hiftory there
are facts prefented to the meditation of the
obferver, which, though confirmed by the
moft convincing teftimony, feem, on the firft
view, to be deftitute of probability. Of this

* Henry IV. P. I. Act iii.
† From the *Journal de Phyfique*, Pluvoife, Year 8.

5 kind

kind is that of people confumed by coming into contact with common fire, and of their bodies being reduced to afhes. How can we conceive that fire, in certain circumftances, can exercife fo powerful an action on the human body as to produce this effect? One might be induced to give lefs faith to thefe inftances of combuftion as they feem to be rare. I confefs that at firft they appeared to me worthy of very little credit, but they are prefented to the public as true, by men whofe veracity feems unqueftionable. Bianchini, Moffei, Rolli, Le Cat, Vicq d'Azyr, and feveral men diftinguifhed by their learning, have given certain teftimony of the facts. Befides, it is more furprifing to experience fuch incineration than to void faccharine urine, or to fee the bones foftened to fuch a degree as to be reduced to the ftate of jelly? The effects of this combuftion are certainly not more wonderful than thofe of the bones foftened, or of the diabetes mellitus. This morbific difpofition, therefore, would be one more fcourge to afflict humanity; but in phyfics, facts being always preferable to reafoning, I fhall here collect thofe which appear to me to bear the impreffion of truth; and, left I fhould alter

the

the fenfe, I fhall quote them fuch as they are given in the works from which I have extracted them.

" We read in the tranfactions of Copenhagen, that in 1692, a woman of the lower clafs, who for three years had ufed fpirituous liquors to fuch excefs that fhe would take no other nourifhment, having fat down one evening on a ftraw chair to fleep, was confumed in the night-time, fo that next morning no part of her was found but the fkull, and the extreme joints of the fingers, all the reft of her body, fays Jacobæus, was reduced to afhes.

" The following extract of the memoir of Bianchini, is taken from the Annual Regifter for 1763 :—The Countefs Cornelia Bandi, of the town of Cefena, aged 62, enjoyed a good ftate of health. One evening, having experienced a fort of drowfinefs, fhe retired to bed, and her maid remained with her till fhe fell afleep. Next morning when the girl entered to awaken her miftrefs, fhe found nothing but the remains of her miftrefs in a moft horrid condition. At the diftance of four feet from the bed was a heap of afhes,

F   in

in which could be diftinguifhed the legs and arms untouched. Between the legs lay the head, the brain of which, together with half the pofterior part of the cranium, and the whole chin, had been confumed; three fingers were found in the ftate of a coal; the reft of the body was reduced to afhes, and contained no oil; the tallow of two candles was melted on a table, but the wicks ftill remained, and the feet of the candlefticks were covered with a certain moifture. The bed was not damaged, the bed-clothes and coverlid were raifed up and thrown on one fide, as is the cafe when a perfon gets up. The furniture and tapeftry were covered with a moift kind of foot of the colour of afhes, which had penetrated into the drawers and dirtied the linen. This foot having been conveyed to a neighbouring kitchen, adhered to the walls and the utenfils. A piece of bread in the cupboard was covered with it, and no dog would touch it. The infectious odour had been communicated to other apartments. The Annual Regifter ftates, that the Countefs Cefena was accuftomed to bathe all her body in camphorated fpirit of wine.

Bian-

Bianchini caufed the detail of this deplorable event to be publifhed at the time when it took place, and no one contradicted it. It was alfo attefted by Scipio Maffei, a learned co-temporary of Bianchini, who was far from being credulous; and, in the laft place, this furprifing fact was confirmed to the Royal Society of London by Paul Rolli. The An-nual Regifter mentions alfo two other facts of the fame kind which occurred in England, one at Southampton, and the other at Co-ventry.

" An inftance of the like kind is preferved in the fame work *, in a letter of Mr. Wilmer, furgeon :—" Mary Clues, aged 50, was much addicted to intoxication. Her propenfity to this vice had increafed after the death of her hufband, which happened a year and a half before, for about a year, fcarcely a day had paffed in the courfe of which fhe did not drink at leaft half a pint of rum or anni-feed-water. Her health gradually declined, and about the beginning of February fhe was attacked by the jaundice and confined to her

* Annual Regifter for 1773, p. 78.

bed.

bed. Though she was incapable of much action, and not in a condition to work, she still continued her old habit of drinking every day and smoaking a pipe of tobacco. The bed in which she lay stood parallel to the chimney of the apartment, the distance from it of about three feet. On Saturday morning, the 1st of March, she fell on the floor, and her extreme weakness having prevented her from getting up, she remained in that state till some one entered and put her to bed. The following night she wished to be left alone; a woman quitted her at half past eleven, and, according to custom, shut the door and locked it. She had put on the fire two large pieces of coal, and placed a light in a candlestick on a chair at the head of the bed. At half after five in the morning, a smoke was seen issuing through the window, and the door being speedily broke open, some flames which were in the room were soon extinguished. Between the bed and the chimney were found the remains of the unfortunate Clues; one leg and a thigh were still entire, but there remained nothing of the skin, the muscles, and the viscera. The

bones

bones of the cranium, the breaſt, the ſpine, and the upper extremities, were entirely calcined, and covered with a whitiſh efflor- eſcence. The people were much ſurpriſed that the furniture had ſuſtained ſo little in- jury. The ſide of the bed which was next to the chimney, had ſuffered the moſt ; the wood of it was ſlightly burnt, but the feather- bed, the clothes, and covering, were ſafe. I entered the apartment about two hours after it had been opened, and obſerved that the walls and every thing in it were blackened ; that it was filled with a very diſagreeable vapour ; but that nothing except the body exhibited any ſtrong traces of fire."

" This inſtance has great ſimilarity to that related by Vicq d'Azyr in the *Encyclopedie Methodique*, under the head Pathologic Ana- tomy of Man. A woman about 50 years of age, who indulged to exceſs in ſpirituous liquors, and got drunk every day before ſhe went to bed, was found entirely burnt and reduced to aſhes. Some of the oſſeous parts only were left, but the furniture of the apart- ment had ſuffered very little damage. Vicq d'Azyr, inſtead of diſbelieving this phæno-

menon,

minon, adds, that there has been many other inſtances of the like kind.

" We find alſo a circumſtance of this kind in a work intitled, *Acta Medica et Philoſophica Hafnienſia* ; and in the work of Henry Bohanſer, intitled *Le Nouveau Phoſphore enflammé*. A woman at Paris who had been accuſtomed for three years, to drink ſpirit of wine to ſuch a degree that ſhe uſed no other liquor, was one day found entirely reduced to aſhes, except the ſkull and extremities of the fingers.

" The tranſactions of the Royal Society of London preſent alſo an inſtance of human combuſtion no leſs extraordinary. It was mentioned at the time it happened in all the journals ; it was then atteſted by a great number of eye-witneſſes, and became the ſubject of many learned diſcuſſions. Three accounts of this event by different authors, all nearly coincide. The fact is related as follows :—" Grace Pitt, the wife of a fiſhmonger of the pariſh of St. Clement, Ipſwich, aged about 60, had contracted a habit, which ſhe continued for ſeveral years, of coming down every night from her bed-room, half-dreſſed,

to

to fmoke a pipe. On the night of the 9th of April 1744, fhe got up from bed as ufual. Her daughter, who flept with her, did not perceive fhe was abfent till next morning when fhe awoke, foon after which fhe put on her clothes, and going down into the kitchen, found her mother ftretched out on the right fide, with her head near the grate; the body extended on the hearth, with the legs on the floor, which was of deal, having the appearance of a log of wood, confumed by a fire without apparent flame. On beholding this fpectacle, the girl ran in great hafte and poured over her mother's body fome water contained in two large veffels in order to extinguifh the fire; while the fœtid odour and fmoke which exhaled from the body, almoft fuffocated fome of the neighbours who had haftened to the girl's affiftance. The trunk was in fome meafure incinerated, and refembled a heap of coals covered with white afhes. The head, the arms, the legs, and the thighs, had alfo participated in the burning. This woman, it is faid, had drunk a large quantity of fpirituous liquor in confequence of being overjoyed to hear that one of her

F 4

daughters

daughters had returned from Gibraltar. There was no fire in the grate, and the candle had burnt entirely out in the focket of the candleftick, which was clofe to her. Befides, there were found near the confumed body, the clothes of a child and a paper fcreen, which had fuftained no injury by the fire. The drefs of this woman confifted of a cotton gown."

" Le Cat, in a memoir on fpontaneous burning, mentions feveral other inftances of combuftion of the human body. " Having," fays he, " fpent feveral months at Rheims in the years 1724 and 1725, I lodged at the houfe of Sieur Millet, whofe wife got intoxicated every day. The domeftic economy of the family was managed by a pretty young girl, which I muft not omit to remark, in order that all the circumftances which accompanied the fact I am about to relate, may be better underftood. This woman was found confumed on the 20th of February 1725, at the diftance of a foot and a half from the hearth in her kitchen. A part of the head only, with a portion of the lower extremities and a few of the vertebræ, had efcaped combuftion.

A foot

A foot and a half of the flooring under the
body had been confumed, but a kneading-
trough and a powdering-tub, which were very
near the body, fuftained no injury. M. Chri-
teen, a furgeon, examined the remains of the
body with every judicial formality. Jean
Millet, the hufband, being interrogated by the
judges who inftituted the inquiry into the
affair, declared, that about eight in the evening on the 19th of February, he had retired
to reft with his wife, who not being able to
fleep, had gone into the kitchen, where he
thought fhe was warming herfelf; that, having fallen afleep, he was wakened about two
o'clock with an infectious odour, and that
having run to the kitchen, he found the remains of his wife in the ftate defcribed in the
report of the phyficians and furgeons. The
judges having no fufpicion of the real caufe
of this event, profecuted the affair with the
utmoft diligence. It was very unfortunate
for Millet that he had a handfome fervant-
maid, for neither his probity nor innocence
was able to fave him from the fufpicion of
having got rid of his wife by a concerted
plot, and of having arranged the reft of the
circum-

circumſtances in ſuch a manner as to give it the appearance of an accident. He experienced, therefore, the whole ſeverity of the law ; and though, by an appeal to a ſuperior and very enlightened court, which diſcovered the cauſe of the combuſtion, he came off victorious, he ſuffered ſo much from uneaſineſs of mind, that he was obliged to paſs the remainder of his melancholy days in an hoſpital."

" Le Cat relates another inſtance, which has a moſt perfect reſemblance to the preceding :— " M. Boinneau, curé of Plerquer, near Dol," ſays he, " wrote to me the following letter, dated February 22d, 1749 :—Allow me to communicate to you a fact which took place here about a fortnight ago. Madame de Boiſeon, 80 years of age, exceedingly meagre, who had drunk nothing but ſpirits for ſeveral years, was ſitting in her elbow-chair before the fire, while her waiting-maid went out of the room a few moments. On her return, ſeeing her miſtreſs on fire, ſhe immediately gave an alarm, and ſome people having come to her affiſtance, one of them endeavoured to extinguiſh the flames with his hands, but they

they adhered to it as if it had been dipped in brandy or oil on fire. Water was brought and thrown on the lady in abundance, yet the fire appeared more violent, and was not extinguished till the whole flesh had been consumed. Her skeleton, exceedingly black, remained entire in the chair, which was only a little scorched; one leg only, and the two hands, detached themselves from the rest of the bones. It is not known whether her clothes had caught fire by approaching the grate. The lady was in the same place in which she sat every day; there was no extraordinary fire, and she had not fallen. What makes me suppose that the use of spirits might have produced this effect is, that I have been assured, that at the gate of Dinan an accident of the like kind happened to another woman under similar circumstances."

" To these instances, which i have multiplied to strengthen the evidence, I shall add two other facts of the same kind, published in the *Journal de Medicine* * The first took place at Aix in Provence, and is thus related by

---

* Vol. lix. p. 440.

Muraire,

Muraire, a furgeon : " In the month of February 1779, Mary Jauffret, widow of Nicholas
Gravier, fhoemaker, of a fmall fize, exceedingly corpulent, and addicted to drinking,
having been burnt in her apartment, M. Ro-
cas, my colleague, who was commiffioned to
make a report refpecting her body, found
only a mafs of afhes, and a few bones, calcined in fuch a manner that on the leaft preffure they were reduced to duft. The bones
of the cranium, one hand, and a foot, had in
part efcaped the action of the fire. Near thefe
remains ftood a table untouched, and under
the table a fmall wooden ftove, the grating of
which, having been long burnt, afforded an
aperture, through which, it is probable, the
fire that occafioned the melancholy accident
had been communicated : one chair, which
ftood too near the flames, had the feat and
fore-feet burnt. In other refpects there was
no appearance of fire, either in the chimney
or the apartment ; fo that, except the fore-part
of the chair, it appears to me that no other
combuftible matter contributed to this fpeedy
incineration, which was effected in the fpace
of feven or eight hours."

5

" The

" The other inftance mentioned in the *Journal de Medicine* *, took place in Caën, and is
thus related by Merille, a furgeon of that city,
ftill alive : " Being requefted, on the 3d of
June 1782, by the king's officers, to draw up
a report of the ftate in which I found Mademoifelle Thuars, who was faid to have been
burnt, I made the following obfervations :—
The body lay with the crown of the head
refting againft one of the andirons, at the diftance of eighteen inches from the fire, the remainder of the body was placed obliquely before the chimney, the whole being nothing
but a mafs of afhes. Even the moft folid
bones had loft their form and confiftence ;
none of them could be diftinguifhed except
the coronal, the two parietal bones, the two
lumbar vertebræ, a portion of the tibia, and
a part of the omoplate ; and thefe, even, were
fo calcined that they became duft by the leaft
preffure. The right foot was found entire,
and fcorched at its upper junction ; the left
was more burnt. The day was cold, but
there was nothing in the grate except two or

---

* Vol. lix. p. 140.

three

three bits of wood about an inch diameter, burnt in the middle. None of the furniture in the apartment was damaged. The chair on which Mademoiſelle Thuars had been ſitting was found at the diſtance of a foot from her, and abſolutely untouched. I muſt here obſerve, that this lady was exceedingly corpulent; that ſhe was above ſixty years of age, and much addicted to ſpirituous liquors; that the day of her death ſhe had drunk three bottles of wine and about a bottle of brandy; and that the conſumption of the body had taken place in leſs than ſeven hours, though, according to appearance, nothing around the body was burnt but the clothes."

" The town of Caën affords ſeveral other inſtances of the ſame kind. I have been told by many people, and particularly a phyſician of Argentan, named Bouffet, author of an eſſay on intermittent fevers, that a woman of the lower claſs, who lived at *Place Villars*, and who was known to be much addicted to ſtrong liquors, had been found in her houſe burnt. The extremities of her body only were ſpared, but the furniture was very little damaged.

" A like

" A like unfortunate accident happened alfo at Caën, to another old woman addicted to drinking. I was affured, by thofe who told me the fact, that the flames which proceeded from the body, could not be extinguifhed by water ; but I think it needlefs to relate this, and the particulars of another event which took place in the fame town, becaufe they were not attefted by a *proces-verbal*, and not having been communicated by profeffional men, they do not infpire the fame degree of confidence.

" This collection of inftances is fupported, therefore, by all thofe authentic proofs which can be acquired to form human teftimony ; for, while we admit the prudent doubt of Defcartes, we ought to reject the univerfal doubt of the Pyrrhonifts. The multiplicity and uniformity even of thefe facts, which occurred in different places, and were attefted by fo many enlightened men, carry with them conviction ; they have fuch a relation to each other, we are inclined to afcribe them to the fame cafe.

" I. The perfons who experienced the effects of this combuftion, had for a long time made an immoderate ufe of fpirituous liquors.

" II. The

" II. The combuftion took place only in women.

" III. Thefe women were far advanced in life.

" IV. Their bodies did not take fire fpontaneoufly, but were burnt by accident.

" V. The extremities, fuch as the feet and hands, were generally fpared by the fire.

" VI. Water fometimes, inftead of extinguifhing the flames which proceeded from the parts on fire, gave them more activity.

" VII. The fire did very little damage, and often fpared the combuftible objects, which were in contact with the human body at the moment when it was burning.

" VIII. The combuftion of the bodies left, as a refiduum, fat fœtid afhes, with an unctuous, ftinking, and very penetrating foot.

" Let us now enter into an examination of thefe eight general obfervations.

" The firft idea which occurs on reading the numerous inftances of human combuftion above related, is, that thofe who fell victims to thofe fatal accidents were almoft all addicted to fpirituous liquors. The women mentioned in the tranfactions of Copenhagen had

had for three years made such an immoderate
use of them that she would take no other
nourishment. Mary Clues, for a year before
the accident happened, had scarcely been for
a single day without drinking half a pint of
rum or anniseed-water. The wife of Millet
had been continually intoxicated; Madame
de Boiseon for several years had drunk nothing but spirits; Mary Jauffret was much
addicted to drinking; and Mademoiselle Thuars, and the other women of Caën, were equally fond of strong liquors.

Such excess, in regard to the use of spirituous liquors, must have had a powerful effect
on the bodies of the persons to whom I allude.
All their fluids and solids must have experienced its fatal influence; for the property of
the absorbing vessels, which is so active in
the human body, seems on this occasion to
have acted a distinguished part. It has been
observed that the urine of great drinkers is
generally aqueous and limpid. It appears that
in drunkards, who make an immoderate use
of spirituous liquors, the aqueous part of their
drink is discharged by the urinary passage,
while the alkoholic, almost like the volatile

G   part

part of the aromatic fubftances, not being fubjected to an entire decompofition, is abforbed
into every part of their bodies.

I fhall now proceed to the fecond general
obfervation, that the combuftion took place
only in women.

I will not pretend to affert that men are
not liable to combuftion in the fame manner;
but I have never yet been able to find one
well-certified inftance of fuch an event; and
as we cannot proceed with any certainty but
on the authority of facts, I think this fingula-
rity fo furprifing as to give rife to a few reflections. Perhaps when the caufe is examined, it will appear perfectly natural. The
female body is in general more delicate than
that of the other fex. The fyftem of their
folids is more relaxed; their fibres are more
fragile and of a weaker structure; and therefore their texture more eafily hurt. Their
mode of life also contributes to increafe the
weaknefs of their organization. Women,
abandoned in general to a fedentary life,
charged with the care of the internal domeftic
economy, and often fhut up in clofe apartments, where they are condemned to fpend

2   whole

whole days without taking any exercife, are more fubject than men to become corpulent. The texture of the foft parts in female bodies being more fpungy, abforption ought to be freer ; and as their whole bodies imbibe fpirituous liquors with more eafe, they ought to experience more readily the impreffion of fire. Hence that combuftion, the melancholy inftances of which feem to be furnifhed by women alone ; and it is owing merely to the want of a certain concurrence of circumftances and of phyfical caufes, that thefe events, though lefs rare than is fuppofed, do not become more common.

The fecond general obfervation ferves to explain the third; I mean, that the combuftion took place only in women far advanced in life. The Countefs of Cefena was 62 years of age ; Mary Clues, 52 ; Grace Pitt, 60 ; Madame de Boifeon, 80 ; and Mademoifelle Thuars, more than 60. The examples prove that combuftion is more frequent among old women. Young perfons, diftracted by other paffions, are not much addicted to drinking ; but when love, departing along with youth, leaves a vacuum in the mind, if

its

its place be not fupplied by ambition or in-
tereft, a tafte for gaming, or religious fervour,
it generally falls a prey to intoxication. This
paffion ftill increafes as the others diminifh,
efpecially in women who can indulge it without reftraint. Wilmer, therefore, obferves,
" that the propenfity of Mary Clues to this
" vice had always increafed after the death of
" her hufband, which happened about a year
before:" almoft all the other women, of
whom I have fpoken, being equally uncon-
fined in their actions, could gratify their attachment to fpirituous liquors without oppofition.

It may have been obferved, that the obefity
of women, as they advance in life, renders
them more fedentary; and if, as has been remarked by Baumé *, a fedentary life over-
charges the body with hydrogen, this effect
muft be ftill more fenfible among old women.
Dancing and walking, which form falutary
recreation for young perfons, are, at a certain
age, interdicted as much by nature as by pre-
judice. It needs, therefore, excite no afto-
nifhment that old women, who are in general

* Effai du Syftême Chemique de la Science de l'Homme.

more

more corpulent and more addicted to drinking, and who are often motionless like inani-
mate maffes, during the moment of intoxication, fhould experience the effects of combuftion.

Perhaps we have no occafion to go very
far to fearch for the caufe of thefe com-
buftions. The fire of the wooden ftove, the
chimney, or of the candle, might have been
communicated to the clothes, and might have
in this manner burnt the perfons above mentioned, on account of the peculiar difpofition
of their bodies. Maffei obferves that the
Countefs of Cefena was accuftomed to bathe
her whole body with fpirit of wine; the vicinity of the candle and lamp, which were
found near the remains of her body, occafioned, without doubt, the combuftion. This
accident reminds us of what happened to
Charles II. King of Navarre. This prince,
being addicted to drunkennefs and exceffes of
every kind, had caufed himfelf to be wrapped
up in cloths dipped in fpirits, in order to revive the natural heat of his body, which had
been weakened through debauchery; but the
cloths caught fire while his attendants were

faftening

faftening them, and he perifhed a victim of his imprudence.

Befides accidental combuftion, it remains for us to examine whether fpontaneous combuftion of the human body can take place, as afferted by Le Cat. Spontaneous combuftion is the burning of the human body without the contact of any fubftance in a ftate of ignition. Nature, indeed, affords feveral inftances of fpontaneous combuftion in the mineral and vegetable kingdoms. The decompofition of pyrites, and the fubterranean proceffes, which are carried on in volcanos, afford proofs of it. Coal-mines may readily take fire fpontaneoufly; and this has been found to be the cafe with heaps of coals depofited in clofe places. It is by a fermentation of this kind that dunghills fometimes become hot, and take fire. This may alfo ferve to explain why truffes of hay, carried home during moift weather, and piled up on each other, fometimes take fire. But, can fpontaneous combuftion take place in the human body? If fome authors are to be credited *, very violent combuftion may be produced in our bodies by nature, and by

* German Ephemerides, Obferv. 77.

artificial

artificial proceffes. Sturmius * fays, that in
the northern countries flames often burft from
the ftomach of a perfon in a ftate of intoxication. Three noblemen of Courland having
laid a bet which of them could drink the moft
fpirits, two of them died in confequence of
fuffocation, by the flames which iffued with
great violence from their ftomachs. We are
told by Thomas Bartholin †, on the authority
of Vorftius, that a foldier, who had drunk
two glaffes of fpirits, died after an irruption
of flames from his mouth. In his third century Bartholin mentions another accident of
the fame kind after a drinking match of ftrong
liquor.

It now remains to decide, from thefe inftances, refpecting the accidental or fpontaneous caufes which produce combuftion. Nature, by affuming a thoufand different forms,
feems at firft as if defirous to elude our obfervation ; but, on mature reflection, if it be
found eafy to prove accidental combuftion,
fpontaneous combuftion appears altogether
improbable ; for, even admitting the inftances

* German Ephemerides, Tenth Year, p. 55.
† Firft Century.

of

of people suffocated by flames from their mouths, this is still far from the combustion of the whole body. There is a great difference between semi-combustion and spontaneous combustion, so complete as to reduce the body to ashes, as in the cases above mentioned: as the human body has never been seen to experience total combustion, these assertions seem rather the productions of a fervid imagination than of real observation; and it too often happens that nature, in her mode of action, does not adopt our manner of thinking.

I shall not extend further these observations on the combustion of the human body, as I flatter myself that after this examination every person must be struck with the relation which exists between the cause of this phænomenon and the effects that ensue. A system embellished with imaginary charms is often seducing, but it never presents a perfect whole. We have seen facts justify reasoning, and reasoning serve afterwards to explain facts. The combustion of the human body, which, on the first view, appears to have in it something of the marvellous, when explained exhibits no-

thing

thing but the utmoft fimplicity : fo true it is, that the wonderful is often produced by effects which, as they rarely ftrike our eyes, permit our minds fo much the lefs to difcover their real caufe.

Some people may, however, afcribe to the wickednefs of mankind what we afcribe to accident. It may be faid that affaffins, after putting to death their unfortunate victims, rubbed over their bodies with combuftible fubftances, by which they were confumed. But even if fuch an idea fhould ever be conceived, it would be impoffible to carry it into execution. Formerly, when criminals were condemned to the flames, what a quantity of combuftible fubftances was neceffary to burn their bodies! A baker's boy, named Renaud, being condemned to be burnt a few years ago at Caën, two large cart-loads of faggots were required to confume the body, and at the end of more than ten hours fome remains of the bones were ftill to be feen. What proves that the combuftion in the beforementioned inftances was not artificial is, that people often arrived at the moment when it had taken place, and that the body was

found

found in its natural state. People entered the house of Madame Boiseon at the time when her body was on fire, and all the neighbours saw it. Besides, the people of whom I have spoken were almost all of the lowest class, and not much calculated to give rise to the commission of such a crime. The woman mentioned in the transactions of Copenhagen was of the poorest condition; Grace Pitt was the wife of a fishmonger; Mary Jauffret, that of a shoemaker; and two other women, who resided at Caën, belonged to the lowest order of society. It is incontestible, then, that in the instances I have adduced the combustion was always accidental, and never intentional.

It may be seen, that a knowledge of the causes of this phænomenon is no less interesting to criminal justice than to natural history, for unjust suspicions may sometimes fall on an innocent man. Who will not shudder on recollecting the unfortunate inhabitant of Rheims, who, after having lost his wife by the effect of combustion, was in danger of perishing himself on the scaffold, condemned unjustly by an ignorant tribunal!

I shall

I shall consider myself happy if this picture of the fatal effects of intoxication makes an impression on those addicted to this vice, and particularly on women, who most frequently become the victims of it. Perhaps the frightful details of so horrid an evil as that of combustion will reclaim drunkards from this horrid practice. Plutarch relates, that at Sparta children were deterred from drunkenness by exhibiting to them the spectacle of intoxicated slaves, who, by their hideous contortions, filled the minds of these young spectators with so much contempt that they never afterwards got drunk. This state of drunkenness, however, was only transitory. How much more horrid it appears in those unfortunate victims consumed by the flames and reduced to ashes! May men never forget that the vine sometimes produces very bitter fruit, —disease, pain, repentance, and DEATH!

*How far are the Acts of the Drunkard to be
palliated ?*

This is a point of great importance in civilized fociety : but it is not the province of
the phyfician to decide with a legal view.
Every human being, who was ever intoxicated,
muft have found, on reflection, that he had
faid and done things which he would have
neither thought of or acted in a ftate of fobriety. The peace of his neighbour has, therefore, required that the drunkard fhould anfwer for his conduct. But it may be afked,
ought a madman to anfwer for his deeds?
Certainly : The man who becomes mad from
immoderate vinous potation muft be amen-
able to law, becaufe that madnefs was of his
own feeking.—Again, it may be faid, that the
drunken man, being as much in a ftate of delirium as any maniac, ought he to be punifhed
for doing what he is unconfcious of? Yes :
But punifhment might be mitigated here, if
it fhall appear that no preconceived malice
had

had prompted him. This is, I think, what lawyers call *mal propense*.—Were a man, during ebriety, to fign a deed, by which he fhould difpofe of his property in an improper manner, to the injury of his family; quere, would fuch a deed be legal? It might be deemed legal; but to me it would appear unjuft to confirm it; becaufe the man never formed fuch a refolution when he was in his fenfes. The acts of the drunkard, in this refpect, ought not to be valid: for this plain reafon, in the fame condition he is not allowed to injure his neighbour, or fociety at large, with impunity; and therefore he ought not to be permitted to injure either his family or himfelf. All debts incurred, or money loft at play, in the ftate of intoxication, ought to be declared *null*, on the lofer appealing in a proper manner when fober. This would prevent the gamefter and fyftematic villain from taking advantage of the honeft man, and would correct fome of the greateft evils in the community.

When a drunken man is lavifh of promifes which he never made when fober;

be

be affured, his kindnefs is not worth your thanks.

When you hear a drunken man boafting of his generofity to his friends; beware, how you receive a favour from that man.

When you hear a drunken man telling family fecrets, whether of his own, or thofe of other people; put that man down for a fool; and take care what you fay in his prefence.

When you hear a drunken man boafting of his favours from the *fex*; be affured, that man has no honour.

When you hear a drunken man bragging of his courage; mark that man a coward.

When you hear a drunken man vaunting of his riches; be affured, he cannot be eftimable for his virtues.

When you hear a drunken man pitying misfortunes which he did not relieve when fober; it is the ftrongeft proof that he poffeffes no goodnefs of heart.

Receive no donations from a drunken man; left he fhould afk them again, when fober.

Avoid the company of a drunkard; for if · he infults you, and you fhould infift on fatif-
faction,

faction, he will plead want of recollection, as apology.

Let the fober man beware of the fociety of drunkards, left the world fhould fay, that he means to take an advantage of their credulity.

CHAP. IV.

The Catalogue of Diseases induced by Drunk-enness.

——— *An anxious stomach well*
May be endur'd ; so may the throbbing head :
But such a dim delirium, such a dream,
Involves you ; such a dastardly despair
Unmans your soul as madd'ning Pentheus felt,
When, baited round Cithæron's cruel sides,
He saw two Suns, and double Thebes ascend.

ARMSTRONG.

THIS head very naturally divides itself into two parts.

SECTION I.

The Diseases which appear during the Pa-roxysm of Drunkenness.

As I have purposely avoided the natural history of wine, and said but little of its chemical qualities ; so I shall not take notice in this place of some diseases, that arise rather from the adulteration of vinous liquors, than the effect of ardent spirit. Of this description

tion is the *colica pictonum*, occasioned by the
nefarious introduction of lead, in order to
correct the acid taste of wines. The first
and most fatal disease of our catalogue is,

Apoplexy *.

The last degree of ebriety is apoplexy; a
privation of sense and motion, while respira-
tion, and the action of the heart and arteries
remain. This disease may be occasioned in
two ways during drunkenness. The powerful
stimulus of alkohol may directly act on the
nervous system, and assail the principle of life.
Or it may induce apoplexy, through the in-
tervention of the sanguiferous system, which,
by being inordinately surcharged and stimulated, may cause such an accumulation of
blood, in the vessels of the head, as to bring
on apoplexy, by compressing the brain, the
source of sense and motion. The first will
most readily be induced by the ingurgitation
of a large quantity of raw or undiluted spirit;
and the last will follow the slower mode of
intoxication, from wine or strong malt liquor.

* Apoplexia Temulenta Sauv. Sp. 3.

When

When fudden death takes place, during drunkenneſs, it muſt be in the manner now defcribed. And when a large quantity of ardent ſpirit is ſwallowed at once, it acts ſo ſuddenly on the ſtomach, and by confent with the whole of the nervous ſyſtem, that the common phænomena of ebriety do not take place. There is no time given for the regular fucceſſion of thoſe feelings and paſſions, which, under the more tardy exhibition of wine, always appear. It approaches at once to the moſt dangerous point; for the man often falls down infenfible, as ſoon as he has finiſhed the draught. Nor, on theſe occaſions, does the countenance ſhew any unuſual ſigns of colour or fulneſs: on the contrary, I have always obſerved the face pale and contracted. Arfenic has feldom been taken in ſuch quantity as to deſtroy life ſo quickly as ardent ſpirit. Indeed that metallic poifon, probably acts by firſt decompounding the organization of the ſtomach; whereas the other more directly affails the vital principle in the nervous ſyſtem itſelf. In ſuch a caſe, medical practice could avail but little; unleſs ſufficient life remained for throwing in warm water, or any

aqueous

aqueous or even milky liquid at hand, to di-
lute the spirit, and facilitate its evacuation by
vomiting. Vomiting in all ſtages of temulency
is salutary. Nature in this points to her own
relief. It is here, as when opium has been
taken in great quantities, whether by deſign
or miſtake; if vomiting comes on there is no
danger.

But in particular habits of body, more than
others, ebriety tends to apoplexy. Phyſicians
have, therefore, marked a condition of body,
under the appellation of the *apoplectic make,*
or form. This form conſiſts, in fulneſs of
blood, a large head, ſhort neck, &c., which,
when joined to advanced age, pave the way
to comatoſe affections. When large quantities
of wine, or ſpirituous liquors, are drank after
a full meal of rich food, in ſuch a habit of
body, there is much danger of apoplexy.
Here the blood-veſſels become diſtended with
an immenſe increaſe of chyle, mixed with vinous ſpirit, and both highly ſtimulating. It
is commonly after the approach of ſleep, that
the drunkard is ſeized with apoplexy, when
the digeſtive proceſs ſends forth a copious
ſupply of blood newly prepared. But the

ſtate

ftate of fleep itfelf at all times favours the acceffion of this difeafe. This may, in part, be
accounted for, from the increafe of power it
gives to digeftion; and in part, to the lefs ex-
panded ftate of the lungs, and diminution of
external ftimuli, by the attention of the fyftem
being paffive. The mechanical effect of an
overloaded ftomach, compreffing the defcending aorta, is alfo faid to have confiderable
fhare, in the production of apoplexy.

The proximate caufe of apoplexy, as appears by diffection, is blood or ferum effufed
into the ventricles of the brain; or between the
dura mater, pia mater, and brain, and the cranium. Thefe, by compreffing the medullary
fubftance and origin of the nerves, caufe the
abolition of fenfe and motion. Among perfons in the habit of bibacity, this kind of
death is frequent: for predifpofition is by that
means acquired. The circulation of the blood
through the fubftance of the brain becomes,
by every fit of drunkennefs, more impeded by
the obliteration of fmall veffels; hardening
and offification of particular parts; while the
finufes and veffels on the furface are unufually
diftended. As drinkers of porter and ale are
most

moſt liable to the *florid* apoplexy, may not this, in a great meaſure, be attributed to the great ſupply of nouriſhing matter which theſe liquors afford ; and to the bitters, and narcotic drugs, which are fraudulently mixed with them, as mentioned before ? The drinker of malt liquor grows fat and corpulent ; while the drinker of ſpirits becomes thin and emaciated.

I have, in the former chapter, ſaid that *purl drinkers* were very liable to apoplexy and palſy. Bitters of all kinds ſeem to poſſeſs a narcotic power ; and, when uſed for a conſiderable length of time, deſtroy the ſenſibility of the ſtomach. This is a claſs of medicines that requires much caution in the treatment of dyſpeptic complaints, what are called weak digeſtion. A celebrated medicine, ſome years ago, for the gout, was offered to the public, under the name of the *Portland Powder* *. It was compoſed chiefly of bitters ; and though it was known to alleviate, or cure the gout, it was always at the expence of the conſtitution : for, in the ſpace of a few months after the arthritic affection diſappeared, apoplexy, palſy, and drop-

* Cullen's Firſt Lines, *Gout.*

ſy,

fy, commenced, and foon proved fatal to the patient. The *purl drinker* is expofed to fimilar danger; and, fooner or later, muft fuffer for his indulgence, by an attack from thofe dreadful maladies. Some people are very fond of *herb-ale*, and *diet drinks*, the ingredients of which are bitter herbs and roots, and are equally pernicious when continued long, or frequently reforted to.

When apoplexy has once affected a perfon, in the advanced period of life, even if temperate in modes of living, it ought to be a *veto* againft the ufe of all fpirituous or fermented liquors. In fuch conditions of body, it is furprifing how fmall a quantity of wine will induce ftupor.—A gentleman of my acquaintance was fubject to *periodical apoplexy*, (for fuch I prefume to call it, from the frequent attacks,) for the laft three years of his life. Such was the recurrence of this difeafe, that certain figns of plethora always indicated an approaching fit. From thefe premifes, I often foretold to his relations the exact period of a new paroxyfm. Some paralytic affection commonly remained after each attack, fuch as hefitation of fpeech, inability to retain his urine

and

and ftools, &c. This gentleman was now upwards of feventy ; and had nothing befides that conftituted the apopleƈtic make : he had been accuftomed to much country exercife ; and always very moderate in the ufe of wine : but now he could not take two glaffes, without defeƈt of voice and fpeech, and ftupor coming on. Yet, in this fituation, he had upwards of thirty diftinƈt fits of apoplexy, the greater part of which I faw, and he died in one of them.

This difeafe being fo frequent an attendant, or a confequence of vinolency, holds up a moft awful warning to the inebriate. The thought of a human being rufhing into eternity, from a board of gluttony, riot, and intemperance, ought to appal the moft depraved and obdurate of mortals!

Epilepfy*, Hyfterics, and Convulfions.

I clafs thefe difeafes together, for obvious reafons, as they nearly acknowledge the fame proximate caufe, and are apt to occur during ebriety, in the fame perfon. It is in the early ftage of temulency that thefe affections chiefly appear; at leaft before much ftupor comes on; and I fufpect they are feldom known but where there is a ftrong predifpo-fition. The ftimulus of vinous fpirit brings forth a large portion of pleafurable fenfation, and induces confiderable mobility of the ner-vous fyftem; and with thefe, great fulnefs and turgefcency of the blood-veffels of the brain. I have known a number of perfons, of both fexes, but particularly feamen, who were fub-ject to epilepfy, and never got drunk without a fit coming on. Two of thefe men, unfor-tunately, fell overboard in that condition, and were drowned at fea.

To thofe of the other fex, who happen to be addicted to the bottle, the hyfteric affection is very apt to occur during the paroxyfm. There are few female drunkards that do not experience this: for, as fine fpirits are eafieft to inflame, fo flight irritations that ruffle the temper, and excite anger, are feldom quieted without fome degree of hyfteric paffion. In feveral cafes, the frequent appearance of this affection has firft led me to detect the unhappy

pro

propenſity. That modeſty which is innate in
the female conſtitution, preſerves them from
indulgence in company; and they are commonly ſolitary dram-drinkers. This delicacy
of feeling, ſometimes carries them great
lengths in concealing their ſituation; and in
making them feign complaints to ward off
ſuſpicion. I have known a medical attendant
acquire much credit from the adminiſtration
of his *catholicon;* when a gentle nap had performed the cure of an indiſpoſition, of which
he had formed no conjecture.—Irregular men-
ſtruation, and abortion, in the early months
of pregnancy, are the frequent conſequences
of inebriation in the fair ſex.

I remember to have ſeen a woman, many
years ago, who was much given to ſpirituous
liquors; and, when intoxicated, was often
ſeized with a convulſive motion in the muſcles
of the lower part of the face, which ſometimes induced a diſlocation of the lower jaw.
Violent emotions of paſſion uſually brought
on theſe convulſions. The common people,
not inaptly, attributed the luxation, as a puniſhment from Heaven for her profane ſwear-
ing, for ſhe became ſilent the moment it took

4   place.

place. The complaint was always remedied at the fhop of a neighbouring furgeon and apothecary.

Oneirodynia * :—*fearful Dreams.*

I know not whether *incubus*, the night-mare, is to be juftly taken into our catalogue. Fearful dreams are, however, common enough towards the decline of the paroxyfm: the ful-nefs of the veffels of the brain, and perhaps alfo the overloaded ftomach, fufficiently ex-plain them. The dream of the officer, who wifhed to fight his friend, as mentioned be-fore, is of this kind : to which ought to be added, the account of the drunken party at Agrigentum, as quoted from Burton, in the laft chapter. Did the memory of drunk-ards ferve, I fufpect, we fhould be furnifhed with numerous curious ftories of a fimilar kind.

The power which the body poffeffes, dur-ing intoxication, to refift *contagion*, and to bear *cold*, is well known : and it might pro-

---

* Ephialtes Plethorica Sauv. Sp. 1.

bably

bably prove a defperate remedy againft fome
difeafes. But it ought to be remembered, that
the exhaufted condition of the body, after
ebriety, as much favours the action of *marfh
effluvium* and *infection*, as the excited condition
repelled it before. It is in this ftate that the
fevers of tropical climates fo readily feize
our feamen and foldiers in the Weft Indies:
the typhous contagion of this country is alfo
extended in a fimilar manner.

SECTION II.

The Difeafes induced by habitual Intoxication.

Phlegmafiæ:—Inflammatory Difeafes.

The difeafes of the inflammatory clafs, are
a frequent confequence of intoxication ; particularly to perfons about the prime of life ; of
vigorous conftitution, a full habit of body,
and eafily fuceptible of ftimuli. How can
this be otherwife? The body, by drinking
fermented liquors, or fpirits, is often excited
to the laft degree: undergoing, in that ftate,
all

all the viciſſitudes of temperature; ſtewed
ſometimes in a hot room; and, at another,
ſtretched along the damp and cold ground, in
the open air, and frequently in the ſevereſt
ſeaſon. It is in this manner that *phrenitis*,
brain-fever, *rheumatiſm*, *pleuriſy*, &c. are to
be accounted for, after a fit of ebriety.

Gaſtritis and *enteritis*, inflammations of the
ſtomach and bowels, are common followers
of the large uſe of ardent ſpirit. It is even
ſurprizing that theſe diſeaſes are not more
often met with from this cauſe. The ſtomach
is a highly ſenſible organ; and in particular
conditions of the ſyſtem, cannot be ſtimulated
to any great degree without partaking more
or leſs of inflammation. Indeed, theſe diſeaſes, in general, are very quickly fatal: they
perform the work of death, in the ſhort ſpace
of a day or two; and with but little warning
to the patient. The pain and heat about the
region of the ſtomach, deceive ſo far, that
freſh quantities of ſpirits are taken down with
a view of relieving a cramp, and thus, in a
manner, fuel is heaped on the fire.

Ophthal-

Ophthalmia :—Inflammation of the Eyes.

This complaint of the eyes is one diſtin-
guiſhing badge of a drunkard; remarked by
the vulgar, as if to point him out to the finger
of ſcorn. Solomon ſays, " Who hath woe?
" who hath ſorrow? who hath contentions?
" who hath babbling? who hath wounds
" without cauſe? who hath redneſs of eyes?

" They that tarry long at the wine; they
" that go to ſeek mixed wine *." The wiſe
king of Iſrael, who knew human nature well,
and probably ſpoke from experience, has, in
this text, given a fine ſummary of the evils
which follow bibacity.

The eye is ſo conſtructed, that it readily
diſcovers, by its turgid veſſels in the *tunica
adnata* or white, the effects induced by a hur-
ried circulation. By theſe means it diſplays
ſome of the moſt obvious phænomena of
drunkenneſs. But the turgeſcence and redneſs of the coats of the eye do not always
ſubſide with the ſolution of the drunken paroxyſm: a true inflammation ſucceeds, attended with pain, intolerance of light, &c.;

* Proverbs, chap. xxiii. 29, 30.

hence

hence specks on the eye, dimness of sight, and other frailties of that organ, are often permanent.

Carbuncles.

Tumors and leprous eruptions, of various size and colour, appear about the nose, and other parts of the face. The vigorous circulation, and determination to the head, may have some effect, in increasing the disposition to these cutaneous affections: but I have some suspicion that they are induced, in a great measure, by the chemical qualities of alkohol, most likely by the evolution of hydrogen in the course of the circulation; and they appear in the face where the superficial blood-vessels are more numerous than in any other part of the body. It is in these vessels that the hydrogen attracts oxygen from the atmosphere; the blood in them becomes preternaturally florid; the skin is thus excited and inflamed, and the spots appear in consequence. Darwin* speaks of them as being sympathetic of diseases of the liver. Although predisposition may much assist here, yet, I think, from what I have observed, that a long use of spirituous

* Zoonomia.

liquors

liquors will caufe the growth of thefe eruptions in any conftitution whatever. There is
no deformity incident to the human body
more difgufting than this. See Shakefpear's
defcription of Bardolph's nofe in the laft
chapter.

Hepatitis :—Inflammation of the Liver.

Hepatic inflammation, both of the acute
and chronic fpecies, is a common effect of
hard drinking. The liver, indeed, more than
other vifcera, appears to be particularly fubject to difeafes from this caufe. The viciffi-
tudes of heat and cold, to which the inebriate
is fo often expofed, may have fome fhare in
the production of this complaint, like other
phlegmafiæ; but the chief caufe muft be the
fpirituous ftimulus. It is not evident whether
the inflammation may be propagated from the
duodenum, along the common and biliary
ducts, to the fubftance of this vifcus; or whether the blood, highly charged with alkohol,
may not be the means of exciting hepatitis.
The chronic fpecies is not a painful difeafe;
is flow in its progrefs, and frequently gives
no alarm till fome incurable affection is the
con-

confequence. It is probable that this inflammation, in fome degree or other, always precedes the enlarged liver, and particularly that form of it that may be properly called the *turbercular difeafe of the liver.*

Podagra:—Gout.

This difeafe, fo often the companion of wealth and indolence, has been fo frequently induced by excefs in love and wine, that in every age it has been juftly ftyled the offfpring of Venus and Bacchus. This fact, I believe, is fufficiently fubftantiated in the records of Medicine; for gout is very feldom or never feen in the habitations of poverty and labour.

Excefs in vinous potation too often gives a ftimulus to the other paffion; but when together they are immoderately practifed, and often repeated, debility of more than a common kind is induced. If there is a hereditary difpofition to gout, all exceffes muft be more hurtful. In youth hard-drinking is particularly injurious; it brings on premature decay; and, more than any other caufe, paves the way for the difeafes of age before the meridian

ridian of life. But as the organs of digeſtion
are ſo principally concerned in gout, the exceſs in drinking acts there with peculiar force.
It is highly probable that the mere pains, and
inflammation of the joints, are very ſecondary
ſymptoms of this complaint; and that the
only ſure way to ward it off is by preſerving
the vigour of the digeſtive organs by temperate and abſtemious living ; and by beginning
early in youth to purſue a regular and active
mode of life. Theſe are the beſt ſecurity for
a ſound conſtitution, which alone can inſure
a happy and healthy old age. It is true, few
young men will ſubmit to ſuch rigid precepts:
and experience of their truth and value is too
often to be purchaſed at the expence of health.
Yet there are many examples to be found, of
men who have ſuffered miſery for years, and
dragged out a wretched exiſtence under arthritic pains, that would gladly forego the pleaſures of wine, had they life again to renew.
As example is therefore better than precept,
the juvenile debauchee ſhould be occaſionally
introduced into the ſick chamber of the hoary
veteran in exceſs. If the children in Lacedæmon were to be trained to temperance, by

I   looking

looking on the difgufting actions and revelry of drunken flaves, let the youths of the prefent time be inftructed from the unwieldy joints, withered limbs, and hypochondriacal glooms of our modern Arthritics.

Schirrus of the Bowels.

Ardent fpirit hardens and contracts the animal fibre, and coagulates the juices. Hence the fenfibility of different organs is gradually exhaufted; and the veffels, whether arteries, veins, lymphatics, or other canals and ducts for conveying fluids, are leffened in their diameter, and ultimately obftructed. A fchirrus of the ftomach, at leaft of the pylorus, and liver efpecially, are frequent concomitants of habitual ebriety*. But the inteftines, pancreas, fpleen, and perhaps the kidneys, are alfo liable to the fame affection; all of which, after a certain time, are incurable, and often fpeedily fatal. The dram and purl drinker may fooner experience thefe evils than other drunkards, but even the guzzler of

* Vide Morgagni De Caufis et Sedibus ubicunque de fectionibus temulentorum differuit.——See alfo Baillie's Morbid Anatomy, Difeafes of the Liver.

*I   fmall-

fmall-beer has no fecurity againft them. Nay, fo fure and uniform is this effect of producing difeafed bowels, by fermented liquors, that in diftilleries and breweries, where hogs and poultry are fed on the fediments of barrels, their livers and other vifcera are obferved to be enlarged and hardened, like thofe of the human body; and were thefe animals not killed at a certain period, their flefh would be unfit to eat, and their bodies become emaciated.

Icterus :—Jaundice.

This difeafe is frequently a confequence of the preceding one, affecting the liver; when, by its enlargement, the biliary veffels and ducts are compreffed, and the free egrefs of the bile prevented; by which means it is, by abforbing veffels, carried into the circulation, and there defœdates the whole body. It is another of thofe difgufting figns which the habit of intoxication gives to the external form: when jaundice appears, it may be reckoned a proof of the patient being a ve-teran worfhipper at the fhrine of Bacchus. In moft cafes, it may be deemed the birth-

right

right of dram-drinking, or the ufe of grog;
but all other liquors produce it by long continuance. Towards the end, the complexion
and eyes, from being yellow, put on a fable
hue, which is a fymptom of approaching dif-
folution. The drunkard fhould be taught to
look into a glafs, that he may fpy the changes
in his countenance : the firft ftage would prefent him with rednefs of eyes; the fecond
would exhibit the carbuncled nofe; and the
third, a yellow and black jaundice. In the
body of the Inebriate, the liver might be juftly
called the *officina morborum** !

Dyfpepfia :—Indigeftion.

There are fo many organs concerned in
the proceffes of digeftion, chylification, and
fanguification, that we cannot be furprifed at
the effects of hard drinking in deranging
them : for the firft introduction of the liquor
into the body comes in direct contact with
moft of them; fuch as the ftomach, inteftines,

---

* Feb. 24. I have at prefent a patient juft recovering
from *difeafed liver and jaundice;* who, by giving up the vinous ftimulus at once, has been miraculoufly fnatched from
the verge of the grave !

biliary

biliary and pancreatic ducts, lacteals, &c.
Want of appetite and bad digeftion are therefore common with drunkards. The ftomach,
next morning after a laft night's debauch, is
left in a ftate of febrile debility; its mufc lar
power feeble and exhaufted; and the gaftric
juice vitiated and unfit to excite the defires of
healthful appetite, or to perform the office of
an active folvent, in the bufinefs of preparing
the food. Hence to make a good breakfaft
has always been reckoned a fign of good
health, and a proof of temperance. The ftomach, by degrees, grows torpid from immoderate ftimuli, and their frequent repetition,
till it feels little inclined to receive that mild
and bland nourifhment which is ufually ferved
up for the morning repaft. In this manner
dyfpeptic complaints firft commence; acidity,
cardialgia, flatulence, and naufea, are fucceeded by nervous irritability, and pain, which
tend to fix the diftrefs of the inebriate. To
relieve thefe, the megrim, *tædium vitæ*, and
hypochondriacifm, which accompany them,
he flies to his bumper. Thus every fucceed-
ing day's potation exceeds its predeceffor in
quantity, and he becomes a habitual drunkard.

I 3   The

The morning hours of such a man, when neither business or rational recreation can engage him, are spent in listless inactivity; he flies from trifle to trifle, expresses his *ennui* by constant yawning, and impatiently counts the tardy hours that shall relieve his longing for the bottle. The man who has once exhibited such symptoms is on the high-road to ruin. I have witnessed the situation of some drunkards, when their potation had been longer withheld than usual; it is impossible to relate such a scene; frantic gestures; hideous yells; screams of torture; looks of despair; groans, sighs, weeping, and gnashing of teeth; are but a describable part of it: it may literally be summed up in what is called the " *torments of the damned.*"

In such cases of dyspepsia, accompanied by these strong mental hallucinations, it is in vain to expect a cure from articles of medicine. The habit of drinking must be abandoned, and moral arguments, with such religious admonitions as inspire hope, must be speedily employed to prevent suicide or derangement of intellect.

Hydrops ;

Hydrops :—Dropsy.

When infractions and enlargements of the abdominal viscera take place, the dropsy, next, makes its appearance. The free return of blood to the heart is impeded; and thus exhalation is increased. But the torpid and palsied state, if I may so call it, of the absorbent system, best explains the accumulation of aqueous fluid in the several cavities. The lymphatic vessels, like the veins and arteries, possess muscular power, by which their contents are propelled. This muscular power, by excessive stimulus, is liable to be exhausted, as in other parts of the body, and the action of the absorbents is thereby lessened. Thus, while an increased proportion of fluid is effused from the relaxed exhalants, the debilitated absorbents are incapable of taking it up. We observe the effect of these vessels being strongly stimulated in the stomach and intestines, by the thirst which succeeds the large ingurgitation of ardent spirit. In the like manner constipation is produced, from the more fluid fœcal matter being absorbed, while the more dry parts of the mass are with difficulty pressed forward. Diseases of the liver,

I 4

more than others, feem to be followed by
hydropic difpofition. I think it requires fomething beyond the mechanical refiftance of
difeafed vifcera to explain this; for that organ, it would appear, poffeffes fome uncommon fympathy or connection with the functions of the lymphatic fyftem. Dropfy is,
therefore, very frequently the harbinger of
death with the inebriate.

Tabes : Atrophia :—Emaciation of Body.

Thefe complaints naturally follow the
weakened condition of the ftomach and ali-
mentary canal. The lacteal veffels themfelves,
by the frequent application of alkohol, are
rendered torpid, conftringed, or impacted;
and the glands of the mefentery, for the fame
reafon, are made impervious. But when the
bile, gaftric and pancreatic juices, are all vitiated
and depraved, how is it poffible that healthful
nourifhment can be prepared? I have feen, in
the fpace of a few months, a man of the
largeft fize, by the immoderate ufe of fpirituous potation, reduced to a mere fkeleton.
Even when fome degree of appetite remains, the food gives no fupport; for it

cannot

cannot paſs into the blood to recruit the deficient juices ; hence emaciation of body and
all its conſequences. A few weeks' indulgence in raw ſpirit, or ſtrong grog, in large
quantity, will induce theſe diſeaſes. Like
many others which follow ebriety, they give
little pain ; and as the mental powers are
lulled into ſtupor the greater part of the day,
the approaches of an incurable malady are not
ſufficiently watched.

Syncope :—Palpitatio.

Fainting fits and palpitation of the heart,
ſometimes accompany exceſſive debility from
habitual bibacity ; and are called nervous
ſymptoms. But the moſt alarming degree of
theſe evils is, when they are the effect of organic affections of the heart, pericardium, and
large blood-veſſels. A hydrothorax, dropſy
of the pericardium, oſſification of the valves
of the heart, coronary arteries, and aorta itſelf, have all been diſcovered by diſſection in
the bodies of men ſubject to temulency *.
The patient commonly dies ſuddenly at laſt,
after being long tormented with anxiety of

* Morgagni, Lib. II. Epiſt. xxvi. 13—37. Epiſt. xxviii.

the

the moſt diſtreſſing kind, frequent fainting
fits, fearful dreams, that make him ſtart from
his ſleep with ſigns of the utmoſt terror and
agitation, and great dejection of ſpirits. To
theſe may he added, thoſe ſymptoms which
conſtitute the " *Angina Pectoris*" of ſome authors. The ſubjects of theſe horrid complaints ſeem to undergo, every hour, all the
pangs of diſſolution. They rank among the
moſt fatal and terrible evils of this gloomy
catalogue.

Diabetes :—Exceſſive Diſcharge of Urine.

The majority of perſons whom I have
known ſubject to diabetes, were lovers of the
bottle. About the proximate cauſe of this
diſeaſe, various opinions have been given by
phyſicians : in this place, therefore, I ſhall be
permitted to refer it to ſome depravity of the
organs of digeſtion. I ſuſpect that many
drunkards have this complaint upon them
without taking notice of it ; and that it comes
and goes, without creating alarm, juſt as they
happen to live regular or otherwiſe. Dr.
Rollo, of the Royal Artillery at Woolwich, has
lately publiſhed an ingenious chemical *Theory*
of

of Diabetes; and his practice has been attested by some striking cases, one of which I attended for a short time. It there appears, that the saccharine urine always followed the use of malt liquors, and such other matter as contained the basis of the saccharine acid : and was cured by a diet in every respect highly animalised, and directly opposite to the articles just mentioned. Hepatic diseases being so common from hard-drinking, and the bile being so important an ingredient in preparing the chyle and the blood, are presumptive proofs, that diabetes may derive much explanation from these sources : but what chemical analysis can unfold the nice operations, and wonderful arcana of Nature!

It is impossible to mention the name of Dr. Rollo, without adverting to the valuable reformations he has effected in the Artillery Hospital at Woolwich. The success of these measures affords a striking contrast to the opposition which I met with in attempting similar improvements in the naval department*.

---

* Vide Med. Nautica; where all the late corrections are detailed, and others pointed out for the information of posterity.

Locked

Locked Jaw.

This difeafe is more frequent in warm than cold climates : it has fucceeded a fit of ebriety when the patient, in the exhaufted ftate, has flept in the open air, or been expofed to the chilly damps of the evening. I think a cafe of this defcription is mentioned by Dr. Girdleftone.

Palfy.

Tremors and paralytic affections are common followers of the *apoplexia temulenta*. The head and hands of fome inebriates, particularly in the morning, fhake and tremble; but regain their ufual ftrength, and become fteady, as the dofe of ftimulus is repeated. Men of this defcription are a kind of living thermometers; as the blood warms, their fpirits rife; and when it cools again, by withholding their dram, they fink into languor and dejection. When affections of this kind make their appearance, the wretched inebriate has almoft finifhed his career of diffipation : the *filver cord* of life is nearly loofed, and the *wheel broken at the ciftern !*

Ulcers.

Ulcers.

When habitual intoxication has fufficiently weakened the folids and polluted the fluids of the body, it alfo excites difeafes of the fkin, that readily run into foul and incurable fores. Inftances of this kind are to be daily met with in private life.

An ulcer, the moft malignant of its kind, on record, during the late war, infefted particular fhips in the Channel Fleet: and commonly affected a large proportion of the crew before the difpofition to it could be overcome. The character of this fore was directly oppofite to that of the fcorbutic ulcer; and what was found a certain cure for fcurvy, had no effect on the Channel fore. The leaft fcratch on the fkin, the puncture of a lancet, the bliftered part, but efpecially fcalds and burns, degenerated into this ulceration, with a rapidity not to be conceived. Large lofs of mufcular flefh from floughs, and caries of bone, were the confequence. A long hiftory of this epidemic ulcer, is given in the fecond and third volumes of *Medicina Nautica.* From a

fair

fair and extensive view of all the facts connected with its production, I have referred
the cause to the *inordinate use of spirituous
liquors*.

Madness and Ideotism.

"Reputation! Reputation! Reputation!
"O! I have lost my reputation! I have lost
"the immortal part, Sir, of myself; and what
"remains is bestial.—Drunk? and speak par-
"rot? and squabble? swagger? swear? and
"discourse fustian with one's own shadow?
"O, thou invisible spirit of wine, if thou hast
"no name to be known by, let us call thee—
"Devil!—I remember a mass of things, but
"nothing distinctly: a quarrel, but nothing
"wherefore.—O! that men should put an
"enemy in their mouths, to steal away their
"brains! that we should with joy, revel,
"pleasure, and applause, transform ourselves
"into beasts!—I will ask him for my place
"again: he shall tell me I am a drunkard!
"Had I as many mouths as Hydra, such an
"answer would stop them all. To be now a
"sensible man, by and by a fool, and pre-
"sently

" fently a beaſt! O ſtrange! Every inordi-
" nate cup is unbleſſed, and the ingredient is
" a Devil *."

Drunkenneſs itſelf, is a temporary madneſs.
But in conſtitutions where there is a prediſ-
poſition to inſanity and iditoiſm, theſe diſeaſes
are apt to ſucceed the paroxyſm, and will
often laſt weeks and months after it. Wounds
and contuſions of the brain and cranium,
with other organic leſions, have a ſimilar
effect. I have known numberleſs inſtances of
theſe kinds of *Mania* † and *Amentia* ‡. In
courts of juſtice we often hear of men, who
are convicted of improper conduct, pleading
for mitigation of puniſhment, from acting
under temporary inſanity. A ſmall quantity
of liquor is apt to derange theſe people : in
ſuch ſubjects the blood would appear to be
over accumulated in the head, or circulates
unequally there, and thus cauſes delirium.
Seamen, who are ſo much expoſed to blows
and wounds of the head, from the nature of
their duty, are very liable to affections of this
kind.

* Shakeſpear, Othello.
† Paraphroſyne Temulenta Sauv. Sp. 1.
‡ Amentia a Temulentia Sauv. Sp. 7.

But

But independent of conftitutional predifpofition, or lefions of the brain, the habit of
drunkennefs will bring on madnefs and ideotifm. They fometimes follow a ftroke of
apoplexy. It is indeed certain, when this
habit has been long indulged, that the ftructure of the brain becomes more or lefs injured.
Morgagni, in his celebrated work, *De Caufis
et Sedibus morborum*, has furnifhed us with
many inftances of the fubftance of the brain
being much altered, as appeared by his diffec-
tions of drunkards. Thefe inftances exhibited
the fame changes from the healthy ftructure,
which are to be found in the brains of maniacs
and ideots. In fome it was found of a much
firmer confiftence than ufual; and in others
more flaccid * : the cerebrum and cerebellum
more foft † : the cerebrum, cerebellum, and
nerves, were all extremely foft ‡ ; the fubftance of the brain was yellow and foft, feemed

---

* Tamen ea firmitudine cerebrum fuit, ut durius ad id
tempus a me diffectum effe non meminiffem.

Lib. i. Epift. viii. 6.
Portio cerebelli flaccida erat, &c.   Lib. i. Epift. ii. 22.
† Cerebrum et cerebellum moliora, &c.

Lib. i. Epift. iii. 6—16.
‡ Cerebrum, cerebellum, et nervi, fumma erant flacci-
ditate, &c.   Lib. i. Epift. v. 11.

cor-

corrupted *: a boney fubftance, and very hard
gypfeous concretions were found, *in oppofito
nervorum thalamo* † *:* the trunks of the arteries
in the meninges, and even their branches,
which extend to the *plexus choroides,* were
much thicker, and harder than natural ; and,
when dried, difcovered a boney difpofition in
different places ‡.

If the fource of fenfe and motion is thus
liable to be affected by fpirituous potation, we
need the lefs wonder at the lofs of the mental
faculties. How juftly, then, may we exclaim,
in the emphatic language of Shakefpear,
" *Every inordinate cup is unbleffed, and the ingredient is a devil!*"

---

* Subftantia cerebri flava ac flaccida quæ corrupta vi-
debatur, &c.   Lib. i. Epift. xi. 6.

† Officulum, vel concretum gypfeum duriffimum, in
oppofito nervorum thalamo, &c.   Epift. xi. 7.

‡ Sed in tenui meningi arteriarum, trunci omnes, om-
nefque item earum rami, iique prefertim, qui verfus
plexum choroidem contendunt, multo erant craffiores
æquo, et duriores, exficcatique offeam pluribus in locis
naturam oftenderunt.   Lib. ii. Epift. xxvii. 28.

K   *Melan-*

Melancholy.

What I have before said on dyspepsia will supersede many remarks that might have been made under this disease. The melancholy of drunkards, I fancy, is seldom or never found without dyspeptic symptoms. Indeed dyspepsia, hypochondriasis, and melancholia, would only appear to be different degrees of the same complaint. Thus indigestion, proceeding from a debilitated condition of the chylopoetic viscera, without nervous affections, may be called simply *Dyspepsia*. But when apprehensions of danger, ill-grounded fears, and low spirits, accompany impaired digestion, the disease may then be named *hypochondriasis*. And when both these affections are present, while at the same time the mental disquietudes arise to derangement of intellect, or delirium, then only would I call the disease *melancholy*. The morning hours of a drunkard, when the bottle has been long withheld, often exhibit the last degree of dejected spirits, which are apt to bring on hallucination of mind. The habit of ebriety
feeds

feeds itſelf. In the abſence of ſtimulus, the ideas have all a gloomy caſt, and every feeling is unpleaſant: there is an aching void, that nothing can fill up but a renewal of the cup; which is no ſooner quaffed than another is deſired: thus by degrees the brain is injured in its ſtructure by violent action, and every ſpecies of delirium is the conſequence.

Impotency, and Abolition of the Sexual Appetite.

There is ſcarcely an organ of the human body that does not, in its turn, receive ſome depravity from habitual temulency. Impotency may be occaſioned here by a paralyſis of thoſe muſcles which are employed in the ſexual intercourſe; but the appetite itſelf is certainly deſtroyed in time: the ſot loſes all feelings of love. The fair ſex ought at all times to ſhow their utter averſion to a drunkard, and to conſider it an inſult when he dares to approach them. This deportment in the female part of ſociety, would be the ſtrongeſt preventive againſt the vice that could be found; for it annihilates all virtu-

ous

ous attachment among the sexes, and is the greatest foe to sentimental love.

With equal justice, the habit of temulency has been said to debilitate the offspring, and produce a puny race. It is a known law in the animal œconomy, that all secreted fluids partake of the vices of the secerning organ. A healthy action is required in every gland, that it may secrete healthy juices. We have seen that the mental functions become deranged, when the brain is injured in its structure. And if this happens, can it be too gross to suppose, that the organs of generation must equally suffer in both sexes, from frequent intoxication; and if offspring should unfortunately be derived from such a parentage, can we doubt, that it must be diseased and puny in its corporeal parts; and beneath the standard of a rational being in its intellectual faculties?—The best antidote against evils of this description in society is early marriage: which, by preserving the body healthful, and the mind pure, gives the best chance of transmitting these qualities to the progeny.—The *sum total* of all the

diseases

difeafes which flow from habitual drunkennefs, is

Premature Old Age.

The wrinkled and dejected vifage, the
bloated and fallow countenance, the dim eye,
the quivering lip, the faultering tongue, *fans
teeth*, the trembling hand, and tottering gait,
are fo many external figns of bodily infirmity :
while weak judgment, timidity, irrefolution,
low fpirits, trifling difpofition, and puerile
amufements, difcover a mind poifoned by the
bowl of excefs, not broke by the hand of
time !

Infants.

If difeafes of fo ferious a nature appear in
adults, from the inordinate ufe of vinous
fpirit, how much more liable muft feeble infancy be to fuffer from the fame. I am
affraid that this is no uncommon obfervation.
It is well known that nurfes, if they can de-
ferve fuch a name, are in the practice of
giving fpirits in the form of punch to young
children to make them fleep. The effect

cannot

cannot fail to be hurtful: such children are known to be dull, drowsy, and stupid; bloated in the countenance, eyes inflamed, subject to sickness at stomach, costive, and pot-bellied. The body is often covered with eruptions, and slight scratches are disposed to ulcerate.

Again, the food of women who suckle their own children is often very improperly selected. The quantity of the milk, not the quality of it, is studied. It is a well-known fact, that this secretion partakes very much of the nature of the diet that is used; that is to say, certain articles pass through the breast unassimilated: vegetables give a more ascescent milk than animal food; but all drinks, containing *ardent spirit*, such as wine, punch, caudle, ale, and porter, must impregnate the milk; and thus, the digestive organs of the babe must be quickly injured. These must suffer in proportion to the delicacy of their texture; and the diseases which flow from this source are certainly not uncommon. Physicians who have prescribed a diet and regimen for nursing mothers, have not sufficiently attended to the hurtful effects of wine

and

and malt liquors. Porter is generally permitted in large quantities on thefe occafions;
a beverage, if there is any truth in our remarks, highly improper and dangerous. It
would be foreign from the nature of this
work, to extend the fubject farther; but it
feemed neceffary to introduce it, in a book
that profeffedly treats of the effects of ardent
fpirits, on the living body.

CHAP.

CHAP. V.

*The Method of correcting the Habit of In-
toxication, and of treating the Drunken
Paroxyfm.*

We curfe not wine : the vile excefs we blame. ARMSTRONG.

FROM what has been faid in the preceding
pages, the importance of this part of my fubject will be readily admitted. A train of difeafes of the moft dangerous nature, at once
deftroying the body, and depraving the mind,
are the certain followers of habitual ebriety.
Amidft all the evils of human life, no caufe
of difeafe has fo wide a range, or fo large a
fhare, as the ufe of fpirituous liquors. When
we fee dropfies, apoplexies, palfies, &c. mul-
tiplying in the bills of mortality, we muft
look to hard drinking as the principal agent
in bringing on thefe maladies. More than
one half of all the fudden deaths which
happen, are in a fit of intoxication; foftened
into fome milder name, not to ruffle the

feelings

feelings of relations, in laying them before the public.

This vice muft have prevailed early among mankind ; and all good legiflators have endeavoured to oppofe its progrefs in fociety. Among the Athenians, by a law of Solon, the magiftrate who became drunk was put to death ; inferior degrees of punifhment fell upon other orders. Drunkennefs was profcribed at Lacedæmon by the laws of Lycurgus : and, to excite horror among the children, againft a vice fo brutal and degrading, the drunken flaves were expofed before them *. The ancient Saracens and Carthaginians drank no wine. The Nervii ufed no vinous liquor, becaufe it made them lazy and effeminate †. Among the Romans the vice was odious : the whole hiftory of this republic does not mention fuch a phrafe, as a habit of intoxication. The women were punifhed capitally if guilty of it : and the cuftom of faluting women is faid to have been introduced, to difcover whether they drank fpirituous liquors. Ebriety is at all times de-

* Plutarch.
† Cæfar de Bello Gallico. Lib. ii. cap. viii.

grading

grading in men; but in women it is difgufting and abominable. The Koran of Mahomet exprefsly denies wine to the Mufulman. —What can Chriftian Britain offer againft thefe authorities?

Drunkennefs prevails more in cold climates than in warm: phyfical caufes may, in a great meafure, explain this. Heat is one of the great fupports of animal life: it beftows on the mental faculties chearfulnefs and vivacity; and the inhabitants of hot countries are obferved to be more gay and volatile than thofe of the northern regions. As heat fupplies abundant ftimulus, the conftitution, therefore, needs lefs excitement from diet. But the fhivering native of Lapland or Labrador, whofe temperature of climate, for a great part of the year, defcends beneath the freezing point, feels an unufual glow and animation from fpirituous potation, which he cannot obtain from his wintry fkies. His atmofphere thus confpires to make him a drunkard: becaufe, when he firft taftes a beverage that imparts chearfulnefs and ftrength; he is not aware that it is the firft ftep to a courfe of indulgence, that muft ultimately impair his health

health, and abridge his underſtanding *. **Dr.** Falconer, in his Eſſay on Climate, ſays, " If " we go from the Equator to the North Pole, " we ſhall find this vice increaſing, together " with the degree of latitude. If we go from " the Equator again to the South Pole, we " ſhall find drunkenneſs travelling ſouth, ex- " actly in the ſame proportion to the decreaſe " of heat."

When ebriety is frequently repeated it be- comes hurtful in proportion to the heat of the atmoſphere. The feveriſh heat which it creates, joined to that of a tropical climate, muſt the ſooner bring on ſome fatal diſeaſe; or more ſpeedily exhauſt the ſtrength of the body by exceſſive ſtimulation. This fact is daily exemplified among European ſoldiers and ſeamen, as well as new-comers, in the Weſt India Iſlands, who, after getting drunk on cheap new rum, expoſe themſelves in the ſun, or in the night ſleep while the heavy dews are falling; and thus become liable to thoſe acute diſeaſes that carry them off in a few days, in deſpite of all medicine. The French ſol- diers and ſeamen, by being more temperate in

* *Vide* Raynal's Hiſt of America.

living

living than Englishmen, suffered less from the
fevers of these regions, in former wars. But
this does not appear to be the case at present
in San Domingo, where Frenchmen have
died in greater proportion than even our
troops, while we possessed that unwholesome
island. It is well known that the modern
armies of France are much addicted to drinking spirits; and many of their greatest victories are said to have been obtained under the
fury inspired by dram-drinking; the spirits
being supplied to the soldiers while engaged,
by women who attended them for that service. This is a species of prowess which our
tars call *Dutch-courage;* and which, I hope,
will never be resorted to by Britons in the
present contest with France.

This vile habit, it appears, was less known
in Britain three hundred years ago than it is at
this time. Mr. Cambden, in his Annals, under the year 1581, has made this remarkable
observation:—" The English, who hitherto
" had, of all the northern nations, shewn
" themselves least addicted to immoderate
" drinking, and been commended for their
" sobriety, first learned, in these wars in the
" Nether-

" Netherlands, to fwallow large quantities of
" intoxicating liquors ; and to deftroy their
" own health by drinking that of others." I
am much afraid that fome later wars in the
fame countries have not greatly encouraged
fobriety. The Roman armies were allowed
only vinegar and water in all their expeditions ; yet with this fimple beverage they con-
quered the world !

It cannot be doubted that the convivial difpofition of the inhabitants of Great Britain
and Ireland, has a ftrong tendency to extend
the habit of ebriety. There is no bufinefs of
moment tranfacted in thefe iflands without a
libation to Bacchus. It prevails among the
Peers of the realm down to the parifh commit-
tee. Thefe convivial parties are a luxuriant
fcyon of a free country ; where all ranks and
degrees of fociety meet to enjoy friendly in-
tercourfe, without the dread of interruption
from a jealous Inquifition, or the domiciliary
vifits of a tyrant's fpies. But they have often
the bad effect of mixing the profligate with
the good, and debauching the fober citizen :
a certain number of bumper-toafts are to be
gulped down on thefe occafions, without dif-
criminating

criminating the weak head and fickly ftomach from the conftant wine-bibber. As the wine fparkles the fpirits mount, and the heart dilates : man is an imitative animal, and quickly affimilates with his affociates. The refolutions that were formed in the cool part of the morning, foon diffolve before the warming influence of a new toaft and a frefh bowl. Thus clubs are formed ; one party begets another ; dinner fucceeds to dinner ; till the man who ftartled once, at a half-pint, now ftaggers home under the load of one bottle more ! *Evoe Bacche !* The man who was focial at firft in his cups, foon becomes convivial, and ends his career as a fot.

It has been afferted, that one of the beft antidotes againft intoxication is, for the fober man to witnefs the actions of the drunkard. With a mind as yet pure and unfullied with debauch, fuch a fight muft be highly difgufting ; and amidft the rigid manners of a Spartan education it might have great weight. But evil communications corrupt good manners : vice, by being often feen, lofes its deformity ; and the beft of young men have become fots from the contagion of example. A drunkard,
reeling

reeling to and fro in the ſtreets, ſeldom eſcapes the inſults and mockery of ſchoolboys. But the ſame boys, when grown up to men, do not always preſerve the ſame hatred and contempt for the practice. The babbling ſot may, for a time, be their ſport and deriſion ; but a frequent view of the object wears off the ſenſibility of the eyes ; and what they once beheld with diſlike, becomes now their friend and aſſociate.

The allegory of the companions of Ulyſſes being transformed into ſwine, is a fine emblem of this degrading habit. The product of the vinous fermentation is not inaptly typified in the following lines of Ovid :

——— miſceri toſti jubet hordea grani,
Mellaque, vimque meri, cum lacte coagula paſſo,
Quique ſub hâc lateant furtim dulcedine, ſuccos
Adjicit.

A modern London porter-brewer, who mixes *opium and coculus Indicus* with his liquor, may be juſtly compared to the ſorcereſs Circe, in thus compounding her charms and hog-transforming cup :·

Quæ ſimul arenti ſitientibus hauſimus ore,
(Et pudet et referam,) ſetis horreſcere cœpi,
Nec jam poſſe loqui ; pro verbis edere raucum
　　　　　　　　　　Murmur :

Murmur; et in terram toto procumbere vultu:
Ofque meum fenfi pando occallefcere roftro;
Collo tumere toris, et qua modo pocula parte,
Sumpta mihi fuerant, illa veftigia feci.
Claudor hara.   OVID. MET. Lib. xiv. Fab. v. vi.

Man, the lord of creation, when by excefs
and debauch he has loft the faculty of reafon,
is not only levelled with the brutes, but feems
to lofe the refpect of inferior animals. The
generous horfe, when mounted by a drunkard,
forgets his wonted fpirit and dignity of mein,
as if afhamed of his burthen. The dog, at
all other times faithful to man, feels his attachment infulted when he follows a ftagger-
ing mafter. There muft indeed be fomething
ftriking in the manner and countenance, between fobriety and drunkennefs; and why
fhould they not be perceived by thefe faga-
cious domeftic animals? Facts are not want-
ing to prove this, which have come under my
own knowledge. A man, returning home at
night when beaftly drunk, was attacked by
his own houfe-dog, that had obferved fuch
a change in his mafter's voice and appearance, that he probably took him for a hog or
a thief. The noife waked the houfehold, who
were too late to fave the flefhy parts of the

leg

leg from being miferably torn.—A gentleman, after getting very drunk in his own houfe with fome jolly companions, went to take the air in his garden, where he was obferved by fome favourite pointers: but, inftead of their ufual careffes, they fet upon him with great fury; and, Acteon-like, he was hunted round his own walks by his own pack. The confequences might have been fatal, had not his fcreams brought his fervants to his af-fiftance.

Ille fugit; per quæ fuerat loca fæpe fecutus,
Heu famulos fugit ipfe fuos: clama.e libebat,
Actæon ego fum, dominum cognofcite veftrum.

OVID.

The reception which the King of Ithaca met with, after a long abfence, from his dog Argo, was very different from that of the two inebriates. Yet Ulyffes was poor, and in rags, at his return: but his countenance was not altered by debauch, or his face and eyes flufhed with wine. From his travels he had acquired much ufeful knowledge, *mores multorum videt et urbes:* for thefe acquifitions the faithful dog feemed to feel a refpect; and he expired with joy at his feet. Had he re-

L   turned

turned intoxicated with the cups of Circe that were drank by his companions, it is probable this friendly animal might have denied his lord and mafter.

But if the habit of intoxication is obnoxious in all men; in the character of the Judge, the Counfellor, and the Phyfician, it is peculiarly criminal. The man that is daily muddled with wine can poffefs no lucid interval, or power of difcernment; he cannot difcriminate between the evidence of right and wrong; and thus he is equally liable to condemn the innocent with the guilty. Solon, in framing the Athenian code, feems to have been aware of this; and another wife man has faid, "It is not for kings to drink wine; " nor for princes ftrong drink: left they " drink, and forget the law; and pervert the " judgment of any of the afflicted *." The fame maxims apply to the duty of the lawyer; if not, the peace of fociety can never be fecure againft evil advifers. But in the phyfician the habit is ftill more dangerous. Other counfellors of mankind have ftated portions of their time for bufinefs, but the acceffions

* Proverbs, chap. xxxi. ver. 4, 5.

of

of difeafe are uncertain, and the phyfician
may be wanted at the moment when his reafon is overwhelmed with wine. If there is
one profeffion more than another, that requires acutenefs of apprehenfion, ferious reflection, or calm contemplation, it is that of
the phyfician ; for every cafe introduces him
to fomething he never faw before. The
world has, at all times, been little fit to judge
of the medical character; becaufe medical
knowledge is almoft infulated from the common obfervation of mankind. But when you
hear it afferted, that fuch a doctor can prefcribe as well drunk as fober, you muft pity
the weak mind that could form the idea; or
confider fuch language as blafphemy in the
face of reafon :—A drunken phyfician is not
worthy to approach the fick-bed of a Hotten-
tot. I mean not to debar the profeffion from
the feftive board ; for, I think, of all men they
ftand moft in need of relaxation, from the
fatigues of bufinefs. Their's is a continued
round among fcenes of pain, forrow, and
death : the man that employs a large part of
the day in the gloom of a fick chamber is en-
titled to all the comforts that are derived from

the

the fociety of the virtuous and good in the domeftic circle; and ought to have his fhare of amufements in the company of the elegant and polite.

The feeds of this difeafe, (the habit of ebriety,) I fufpect, like many others, are often fown in infancy. I do not merely allude to the moral education. In the prefent ftage of fociety, human kind are almoft taken out of the hands of Nature: and a cuftom called *fafhion*, a word which ought to have nothing to do with nurfing, now rules every thing. The early ftages of our exiftence require a mild bland nourifhment, that is fuited to the delicate excitability of a tender fubject. But it too often happens that the infant is deprived of the breaft, long before the growth of the body has fitted the ftomach for the reception of more ftimulant food. Inftead, therefore, of its mother's milk, the infant is fed on hot broth, fpiced pudding, and, perhaps alfo, that enervating beverage tea. The tafte is thus early vitiated, the ftomach and bowels frequently difordered; and, to add to the mifchief, the helplefs child is forced to gulp down many a naufeous draught of medicine,

or

or bitter potion, that its unnatural mother may
acquit her confcience of having done every
thing in her power to recover its health.
Dyfpeptic affections are in this manner quickly induced : a conftant recourfe to medicine,
wine, cordials, and fpirits, muft be the confe-
fequence; and the child of the fafhionable
lady becomes a certain *annuity* to phyfic; a
drunkard at twenty, and an old man at thirty
years of age. Parents and guardians would
do well to calculate the effects of an appetite,
early accuftomed to ftimulating food; and endeavour to prevent future bad habits, by fuit-
ing the nourifhment to the period of life.

It may now be afked, at what age ought a
child to begin the ufe of wine? To this I
muft reply, that fpirits, wine, and fermented
liquors of all kinds ought to be excluded from
the diet of infancy, childhood, and youth.
Natural appetite requires no fuch ftimulants.
Human blood, and healthful chyle, do not acknowledge *alkohol* to be an ingredient in their
compofition. The ufe of thefe liquors is
hurtful in proportion to the tender age in
which it is begun. The laborious ruftic, whofe
chief beverage is water, or milk, toils through

the

the feafons, is never troubled with dyfpeptic
complaints; and never fuffers from low fpirits
or hypochondriacal apprehenfions. Why,
then, will the better orders of life, lay the
foundation in infancy, for what are to be
conftant troubles to their children while they
live?

When wine was firft introduced into Great
Britain, in the thirteenth century, it was confined to the fhop of the apothecary: it would
have been well had it been ftill confined
there: but fpirituous liquors are not mentioned at that period of our hiftory. They
were probably unknown till our army went
to affift the Dutch in obtaining their inde-
pendency. As an article in medicine the virtues of wine are fovereign in their kind:
there are fome difeafes for which it is the beft
remedy, witnefs typhus fever. But the mind
that leans upon it for fupport under afflic-
tions, trufts to a broken reed, a falfe friend,
a deception that lulls it into fatal fecurity.
The evils and misfortunes of human life muft
be borne with fortitude of a different kind,
and oppofed with religious and moral fenti-
ments. Thefe opiates of the foul do not terminate

minate their operation by increafing the
gloom, and inducing a feverer paroxyfm at
its next recurrence. A man who gets drunk
to forget care, fhould be reminded of the horror that will inevitably follow intoxication, on
the firft return of fobriety.

I am of opinion, that no man in health can
need wine till he arrives at forty. He may
then begin with two glafles in the day : at
fifty he may add two more; and at fixty he
may go the length of fix glafles *per diem*, but
not to exceed that quantity even though he
fhould live to a hundred. Lewis Carnaro, the
Venetian nobleman, who lived upwards of a
hundred, ufed fourteen ounces of wine in the
day. The ftimulus of wine is favourable to
advanced age. The circulating fyftem, after
we pafs the meridian of life, becomes lefs vigorous : and the paffions that formerly added
force and ftrength to the bodily movements,
decline, and are lefs exciting. As the feelings
and fenfibility, therefore, grow blunted and
dull, we can bear, not only with impunity,
but with advantage, thofe excitors that would
have done harm before. Wine, and all fermented liquors, by quickening the circulation

L 4

of

of the blood, generate heat: and it is well
known that increafe of temperature is favourable to old age: heat ftimulates the withered
limb to motion, foftens the rigid fibre, and
opens the dry fkin by augmenting the per-
fpirable fluid. Thus aged people feel additional comfort in warm feafons and climates;
and generally die in fome of the winter
months. For thefe reafons, wine has been
aptly called the " *milk of old age.*"

> O! feldom may the ftated hours return
> Of drinking deep! I would not daily tafte,
> Except when life declines, even fober cups,
> Weak withering age no rigid law forbids,
> With frugal nectar, fmooth and flow with balm,
> The faplefs habit daily to bedew,
> And give the hefitating wheels of life
> Gliblier to play. But youth has better joys:
> And is it wife, when youth with pleafure flows,
> To fquander the reliefs of age and pain?
>
> ARMSTRONG, Art of Preferving Health.

In thofe families where gout and dyfpeptic
complaints are hereditary, the ufe of wine,
and all other fermented liquors, ought to be
cautioufly guarded againft in childhood and
youth. The parent who offers them to the
infant, whatever may be the motives of ten-
dernefs, ought to weigh the confequences. If
the

the babe were left to the inftincts of nature
thefe articles would be the very laft it would
fix upon. Their qualities are fo diametrically
oppofite to the mother's milk. The pleafure
which they afford is momentary; and every
time they are reforted to, there is danger of the
quantity being increafed: of the evils which
refult from this practice there is no end. The
child that is born of gouty and dyfpeptic
parents, ought from its birth to be confined to
the mildeft food; it ought to fubfift on milk
alone as long as poffible: it muft never tafte
wine, even diluted to the utmoft, or beer of
the weakeft kind. Animal food, and broth
made from that, light puddings, and different
articles of cookery where milk forms the chief
ingredient, will extend the diet as the child
grows up; and thus will be laid the foundation of a healthy conftitution, and a temperate
life. It is a contrary treatment that enfures
the approach of thefe maladies; and early
gout is often fixed before the man arrives at
thirty. Such are the baneful effects of early
bad cuftoms; for when the tafte is once confirmed, whether for hot or cold articles; fubftances fweet or four, mild or acrid, they
become

become so interwoven with habit, that we strive in vain to correct them. The late Dr. Cullen, in his Lectures, used to mention a family, all of whom were in the habit of taking a dram at a certain hour before dinner, about one o'clock. When the Doctor expressed his wonder at the practice, it was acknowledged by all, that if the time passed, or if they were from home, and did not get the usual dram, it was attended with a considerable *sense of consciousness*. In plain English, they had got into a very bad habit, and found themselves low-spirited for want of their cordial. This morning dram was probably inculcated by the example of some dyspeptic mother, or an arthritic father. The venerable Professor did not inform us of the future history of this odd family; but I could almost venture to pledge myself, that the whole of them turned out to be drunkards. Indeed where the members of a family were so early initiated into pernicious customs by both precept and example, parents have no right to look for a regular life among their children. In this habit, as in all others, imitation has its powerful effects; and the man is spoiled

in

in the arms of his nurse, while yet an infant.

Some intemperate men, it may have been remarked, have lived to a great age. That some drunkards have numbered eighty years and upwards, there can be no doubt. But what kind of life has that been ? half the time muſt have been ſpent under the impreſſion of deranged intellect ; and their ſober moments, if they had any, muſt have been a continued repetition of mental diſquietudes, dejected ſpirits, and gloomy apprehenſions. If, however, we admit that one drunkard now and then may exceed three ſcore years and ten, the balance is much on the other ſide, when many thouſands fall victims to the bottle before they arrive at thirty. Let the man of reflection only look round him in ſociety ; and as he ſees his acquaintance fall off by the diſeaſes mentioned in our catalogue ; if he has been converſant with the modes of living among theſe perſons, he will find that intemperance in drinking has had a large ſhare in bringing them to the grave.

But it is not drinking ſpirituous liquors to the length of intoxication only that conſtitutes intem-

intemperance. A man may drink a great
deal, pafs a large portion of his time at the
bottle, and yet be able to fill moft of the avo-
cations of life. There are certainly many
men of this defcription, who have never been
fo transformed with liquor as to be unknown
to their own houfe-dog, or fo foolifh in their
appearance, as to be hooted by fchool-boys,
that are yet to be confidered as intemperate
livers. Thefe fober drunkards, if I may be
allowed the expreffion, deceive themfelves as
well as others; and though they pace flowly
along the road to ruin, their journey termi-
nates at the fame goal, bad health. They are
commonly men of eafy difpofitions, and an
indolent turn of mind; like the man whom
Horace defcribes,

—— qui nec pocula veteris Maffici,
Nec partem folido demere de die
Spernentem.

Of the quantity of liquor which fome inebriates are capable of confuming, we have
no accurate accounts. To a certain length,
habit may enable a man to devour an enor-
mous load: but we even fee habitual drunkards in their decline, unequal to their former
quantity.

quantity. Their ſtomachs may ſtill be able to retain it, but the head grows too weak to carry it. The organization of the brain has been injured. The blood-veſſels there become ſtraitened in their capacity to receive blood; ſome are obliterated; while others are uncommonly dilated and diſtended: the ſubſtance of the brain alſo undergoes changes, becomes dry and harder; or ſoft and more flaccid than natural. To theſe may be added, boney, or ſtoney concretions in different places of that organ; effuſions under the cranium, and water in the ventricles. Theſe leſions would ſeem to aſſiſt a ſmaller quantity of liquor in raiſing delirium, and for obvious reaſons. I have heard it aſſerted that ſome coal-heavers and porters in London, will conſume four gallons of ale or porter in the twenty-four hours. This quantity could not be long continued. I knew a marine, in a king's ſhip, who uſually drank four gallons of beer in the day; but he ſoon grew bloated and ſtupid, and died of apoplexy. Among the numerous deaths from intoxication which have come under my own obſervation, or reported to me by ſurgeons, no ſeaman ever exceeded

I

ceeded the bottle of spirit; whether rum of the common strength or malt spirit, made in England, the most fiery of the whole. An officer of the hospital ship of the fleet, besides his allowance of wine, at the mess-table, usually drank a bottle and a half of gin in twenty-four hours. His face, at times, was equal to Bardolph's, with bloodshot eyes, fetid breath, &c. He died of apoplexy and diseased liver. A midshipman of my acquaintance, only sixteen years old, drank in the West Indies, three gallons of punch daily. The ship did not remain long in the country: but he became a professed drunkard, and died lately in the Mediterranean. The following narrative may serve as an example of what is frequently done by a labouring man in an American town, who passes for a *sober citizen*. The daily quantity of spirits (bad rum) consumed by one of these persons, is as follows:

Before breakfast	2 gills.
Before dinner	3
By the time the day's work is done	3
Total	8 gills or 1 quart;

besides

befides what he drinks in porter-houfes, clubs, and other meetings in the evening. The reporter admits that this practice proves fatal, but he does not fay in what length of time, or what difeafes are the fequel. If a fober American labourer can devour this quantity of fpirit, what portion conftitutes a drunkard in that country? It is well that America receives her population from the old continent, otherwife her peafantry muft foon die out. This account is taken from the Medical Repofitory of New York: it furnifhes a fhocking fpecimen of the morals of the lower orders of fociety in the northern provinces of the new world.

How far the rapturous effufions of poets, in the praife of wine, have tended to meliorate or deprave the moral character, may not be the province of a phyfician to difcufs. I am ignorant of what ftupendous works of genius have been planned by fancy, " *in a fine frenzy rolling*" over the fumes of wine. I rather fufpect that fuch buildings may be compared to caftles in the air. Thus a great name of the prefent day, whom this country looks up to, fpoke of the deliverance of Europe

rope from the horrors of the French Revolution with all the confidence of a prophet, who could look into the womb of time. He is ftyled, by way of eminence, " a three-bottle man." But if it was under the influence of that quantity that he planned fo many unfuccefsful expeditions againft the enemy, as a lover of my native land, I cannot help wifhing that this great drinker had been confined to three bottles of water till he had fulfilled his promifes to his countrymen.

Anacreon and Horace, who detail with fo much pleafantry their convivial hours, have fhewn us but one fide of the picture: the fchirrous liver, and the palfied limb, with all the namelefs ills which the body fuffers, before thefe mortal diftempers appear, are thrown into the back ground. Yet the authority of fome phyficians may be quoted in fupport of the lively fallies of thefe poets. Dr. Haller, a man alike famous for his piety and learning, fays, " Ingenium quod excitat vinum, ex " eo clariffime intelligitur, quod ad poefin, " quæ res ingenii eft, mirifice difponat. Per- " petuo ab antiquitate creditum eft, et ipfa " res docet, vini calorem, poetarum furorem,

" et

" et impetum excitare : et Bacchi et Apolli-
" nis furorem unum esse eundemque : quam-
" obrem Ovidius vino carens, in exilio de se
" conqueritur ;

> " Impetus ille sacer, qui vatum pectora nutrit,
> " Qui in nobis esse solebat, abest *."

Hoffman expresses himself much to the
same purpose : " Tam observamus omnes
" hos populos qui vino utuntur, longe ingenio-
" siores esse reliquis hominibus. Nullibi enim
" artes liberales, et disciplinarum studia melius
" floruerunt ac florent, quam dictis in locis :
" vina enim fovent vires, pituitam attenuant,
" mordaces curas humanis mentibus infestas
" abstergunt, vim animo reddunt, spirituas-
" centiam sanguinis provovent, ingeniumque
" accuunt : unde non inepte vinum poetarum
" equus dictum est †." The language contained in these quotations, in my opinion, is more becoming the poet than physician. Poetry, the first of the fine arts, took
its rise among shepherds in the early ages of
society, when the manners of mankind, as
well as their diet, were simple ; when the

* Physiol. lib. xvii. sect. 1—13.
† Hoffm. De Temperamento.

fermen-

fermentation of the juice of the grape was unknown, and when the vine itfelf, either fprung up fpontaneoufly, or was only culti-vated as a fruit-tree. Sentiments of the kind, with thefe phyficians, we imbibe with our claffical education; and we preferve them through life on account of the elegant tafte and language in which they are written. But when we come to engraft them on the ufeful affairs of the world, they elevate the mind above the realities around it, and give a dangerous bias to the moral cha-racter.

A modern Britifh phyfician of great emi-nence, himfelf a poet, far above mediocrity, both in his medical and metrical works has held a language very different from both Haller and Hoffman. He probably carries his antipathy to vinous potation too far; and attributes effects to it that are generally over-charged, if not incorrect *. He was no wine-bibber, and died lately about the age of fe-venty. But I have been told by a lady of great literary and fcientific accomplifhments, who had lived for weeks in the family, that

* Zoonomia.

he

he was rather a grofs eater, and made amends
for the want of vinous ftimulus, by confuming large quantities of animal food. The
mufe of Darwin therefore received no infpi-
ration from Bacchus, in finging the " tiny
" graces" of the plants,

To woo and win their vegetable loves. Bot. Garden.

As far as my own experience goes in re-
forting to wine againft the fatigues of bufinefs, I think, if circumftances were fairly
weighed, they do not much fupport the practice. I have always had more inclination
than opportunities for ftudy. In the practical duties of medicine I have, without pre-
judice, formed my obfervations at the fick-
bed ; and no phyfician ever encountered
more anxiety for the fate of his prefcription,
or felt more fincerely for the recovery of his
patient. My labours in fome periods of the
naval fervice, in point of mental and bodily
exertion, have not been furpaffed by any
member of the profeffion ; nor has the leaft
of thefe been my endeavours to roufe the
apathy and torpid indifference to the fubject
of health in the navy, that pervades the pub-

M 2

lic

lic offices in this country. A great part of my life has been spent among men who are, from situation, said to be much addicted to ebriety: but in the present day, in this respect, naval officers, for sober living, are equal to any other description of persons. My whole experience assures me, that wine is no friend to vigour or activity of mind: it whirls the fancy beyond the judgment, and leaves body and soul in a state of listless indolence and sloth. This is confirmed by what I have observed of the habits of life among some great men whom I have had the honour to number as friends. The man that, on arduous occasions, is to trust to his own judgment must preserve an equilibrium of mind, alike proof against contingencies as internal passions. Even the physician requires this fortitude as much as any individual. He must be prompt in his decisions; bold in enterprize; fruitful in resources; patient under expectation; not elated with success, or depressed with disappointment. But if his spirits are of that standard as to need a fillip from wine, he will never conceive or execute any thing magnanimous or grand. In a survey

vey of my whole acquaintance and friends, I find that the *water-drinkers* poffefs the moft equal temper and cheerful difpofitions. But this does not exclude the temperate ufe of wine, which certainly is lefs in quantity than people commonly imagine.

With refpect to labour of body the fame arguments apply. Vinous liquors for a while increafe mufcular ftrength ; but to a certainty bring on premature wearinefs and fatigue, with more inclination to fleep. Spirits have the fame effects in a greater degree, and caufe a greater confumption of pure air. In a warm feafon or climate, the beft articles to ufe under fevere corporeal hardfhips are the acid fruits, fuch as the lemon and orange, apple, &c. ; or in their want, vinegar and water, as practifed by the Roman foldiers. In winter, plain diet, with a due admixture of animal food, and moderate exercife, are the fure fecurity of preferving warmth of body. Spirituous liquors, though generally practifed, give but a temporary glow, and in the end render the effects of cold more fpeedily hurtful.

A cuftom has long prevailed in this country of drinking wine while at dinner ; this is down-

right

right pampering, and vitiates taſte and healthful appetite. But if there is a gueſt at table who loves his bottle, it affords him an opportunity of getting drunk before the cloth is taken off, to the great annoyance of the company. This cuſtom ought to be pro-ſcribed: " *Thracum eſt.*"

A nobleman of my acquaintance, a flag-officer, a man of the moſt equal temper, who excelled in the mathematical ſciences, was ſubjeċt to hereditary gout; which, by a tem-perate regimen, and the ſpare uſe of wine, he kept under till he was nearly ſixty. After this he was ſeldom without an annual attack; but which did not impair his general health, or deprive him of exerciſe. During a tre-mendous gale of wind in the month of Fe-bruary, while he ſuffered great anxiety for the ſafety of his fleet, he was much expoſed to cold, and was ſeized with a ſevere gouty paroxyſm, which laſted many weeks, and left conſiderable lameneſs behind, as well as ge-neral debility. From habitual coſtiveneſs he had taken Glauber's ſalts as a laxative for twenty years; and his wine, a glaſs or two, always largely diluted. My opinion was, that a more ſtimulating plan was neceſſary;

4   that

that the cold purgative fhould be changed, and generous wine freely indulged. My advice was overruled by thofe who had long attended him, who faid that it was impracticable to alter fuch long habits; and he declined from that moment. In this cafe, wine, that was wifely withheld during the vigour of youth, would now, in old age, and under debility increafing, have been a certain remedy. A life fo valuable ought to have been fpun to its laft thread! Frail indeed is that art whofe profeffors are jealous to have their merits tried by the laws of common fenfe.

There can be no doubt that many perfons have to date their firft propenfity to drinking to the too frequent ufe of fpirituous tinctures as medicines, rafhly prefcribed for hyfterical and hypochondriacal complaints. There are patients who are continually craving after medical novelties, and are in the practice of taking every article that is warming and cordial. People accuftomed to drink very ftrong tea, particularly thofe who indulge in the fineft greens, run great hazard of falling into the fame evil habit. Tea, in the prefent day, has a large fhare in the production of ftomach

M 4   complaints,

complaints, and thofe affections ufually called *nervous*. It powerfully ftimulates the digef-tive organs for a while, and exhilarates the fpirits; but a proportional debility and de-jection of mind fucceed, till, like the dram, it muft be made ftronger and ftronger, and is then followed by a train of dyfpeptic fymptoms, fuch as gaftrodynia, acidity, fla-tulence, hyfterics, barrennefs, and all the evils which flow from a deranged nervous fyftem. Souchong tea, ufed once a-day, made not too ftrong, with a due admixture of cream and fugar, is a harmlefs and agreeable beverage. But hyfon, and all the greens, are powerful narcotics, that deftroy the ftomach; and when a train of ftomach complaints is once fixed, and continued by the ufe of tea, there is no perfon proof againft the temporary eafe which is obtained by fpirituous potation, but whofe permanent effects are difeafe, pain, derangement of intellect, a miferable exift-ence, or premature death. There are cer-tainly many well-meaning people who take frequent drams to relieve uneafinefs of fto-mach, without at all fufpecting that they are doing any thing wrong. When complaints

arife

arife from this habit, they very little confider their daily cordial as the caufe of the mifchief, and too often continue it till the breach in their health is irreparable.

There is another cuftom not uncommon in fome families, but particularly at feafts and entertainments, the ceremony of handing cordials round in the time of dinner, which is againft all rules of temperance. It is deceiving the unwary: for I am fure there are many who drink of thefe *liqueurs* that would blufh to tafle brandy. Yet they are nothing more than brandy difguifed. Many of thefe cordials are impregnated with narcotic fubftances, which add to the noxious qualities of the fpirit. We are told by Dr. Mortimer, in the Philofophical Tranfactions, that a man and his wife died paralytic, who drank daily a dram or two of brandy in which laurel-berries were infufed *. The *liqueur* called *Noyau*, which is imported in greateft perfection from Martinique, is nearly allied to this, having all the flavour of the laurel-bitter, and may be readily imitated by bitter almonds. As the habit of ebriety is fo

* Reid and Gray's Abridgement, vol. vi. p. 270.

difficult

difficult to be overcome, from whatever caufes it began, fo the beft maxim is, " *obftare prin-* " *cipiis*."

However feducing the love of inordinate drinking may be, like other bad habits, mankind feldom get into it at once. There is a gradation in the vice. When the drunkard feels himfelf falling as it were in the fcale of being, he forfakes his former friends, feems to fhun his honourable acquaintance, and flides by degrees into the company of men whom he lately defpifed. Some ftruggles of fenfibility, fome compunctious vifitings, cannot fail to attend fuch a tranfition. A few years ago I met an old and once valued friend in a public walk: being fhort-fighted I did not perceive him for fome time, and he made no advances to fpeak to me. I obferved him more flovenly in his drefs than ufual, and his face rather bloated: I requefted the favour of his company to dinner, which he accepted in an embarraffed manner, and came. But alas! *quantum mutatus ab illo!* At dinner his converfation was all in broken fentences; his fine literary tafte was gone; and the feaft of reafon and the flow of foul had

no

no fhare in our entertainment. He drank inceffantly of fherry, as if infenfible why he did it, and filled bumpers every time. I was called out of the room on duty, but before I returned he had finifhed another bottle of wine.—It is painful to add, in a few weeks he was confined in a mad-houfe! I could trace no caufe for the pernicious habit in this accomplifhed young man but the effect of a proud fpirit broken by difappointments in his profeffion.

When ebriety has become fo far habitual that fome difeafe appears in confequence, the phyfician is for the firft time called in, and a tafk the moft ungrateful devolves upon him. If friends and relations had taken the alarm before to fave the conftitution of the patient, it will at once be found that their attempts proved unfuccefsful. Whatever this difeafe may be, whether ftomach complaints, with low fpirits, premature gout, epilepfy, jaundice, or any other of the catalogue, it is in vain to prefcribe for it till the evil genius of the habit has been fubdued. On fuch an occafion it is difficult to lay down rules. The phyfician muft be guided by his own
discretion:

discretion: he must scrutinize the character
of his patient, his pursuits, his modes of
living, his very passions and private affairs.
He must consult his own experience of human nature, and what he has learned in the
school of the world. The great point to be
obtained is the confidence of the sick man;
but this is not to be accomplished at a first
visit. It is to be remembered that a bodily
infirmity is not the only thing to be corrected. *The habit of drunkenness is a disease
of the mind.* The soul itself has received
impressions that are incompatible with its
reasoning powers. The subject, in all respects, requires great delicacy and address;
and you must beware how you inveigh
against the propensity; for the cravings of
appetite for the poisonous draught are to the
intemperate drinker as much the inclinations
of nature for the time, as a draught of cold
water to a traveller panting with thirst in a
desart. Much vigilance will often be required in watching these cravings; for they
are sometimes attended with modes of deception, and a degree of cunning, not to be
equalled. Nay I have known them employ
force

force in the rudest manner in order to gratify their longing after spirituous liquors. I firmly believe that the injudicious and ill-timed chastisement of officious friends have driven many an unfortunate inebriate to ruin, that might have been reclaimed by a different treatment. Nay, if such corrections are applied when the mind is ruffled with nervous and hypochondriacal feelings, and depressed with low spirits, which so frequently follow a last night's debauch, the consequences may be fatal; and it is well known that suicide has sometimes been first resolved upon after these ghostly admonitions.

When the physician has once gained the full confidence of his patient, he will find little difficulty in beginning his plan of cure. I have on several occasions wrought myself so much into the good graces of them, that nothing gave them so much alarm or uneasiness as the dread of declining my visits after they had been argued out of the pernicious practice. This confidence may sometimes be employed to great advantage when your regimen is in danger of being transgressed, for frequent relapses, and promises

repeatedly

repeatedly broken, will, in such situations, render the physician's visits a work of great trial to his patience. This disease, I mean the habit of drunkenness, is like some other mental derangements; there is an ascendancy to be gained over the person committed to our care, which, when accomplished, brings him entirely under our controul. Particular opportunities are therefore to be taken, to hold up a mirror as it were, that he may see the deformity of his conduct, and represent the incurable maladies which flow from perseverance in a course of intemperance. There are times when a picture of this kind will make a strong impression on the mind; but at the conclusion of every visit, something consolatory must be left for amusement, and as food for his reflections.

It has been a doubt with some physicians, whether even, if the patient were willing, it is proper all at once to leave off wine or spirits. The body being long accustomed to this stimulus cannot be deprived of it, without sustaining manifest injury. This mode of reasoning is founded on the observation that habit has a powerful influence over many

of

of the actions of the animal econ ...; it becomes a part of our nature, and some important operations of the living system are entirely governed by it. The general fact being admitted, it does not follow that such long continued stimuli as have a tendency to destroy the functions of the body, should not, all *at once*, be laid aside. Let us suppose a person for years living in a dungeon, unwholesome and unventilated, till diseases appear from these causes, would any rational being hesitate a moment to bring forth the squalid sufferer into the light of day, that he might have the full benefit of a pure atmosphere? The case is exactly in point; the confined person has been breathing poison, and the drunkard has been swallowing it; he has drank poisonous spirit till it has brought him to the verge of the grave, and yet it is held dangerous to take it away. The practice of physic is sometimes so tightly laced in its technical habiliments that it is incapable of turning round! But it does not appear that ever the living body could accustom itself, strictly speaking, to the use of *alkohol.* The habit of intoxication belongs

to

to the mind. The nature of the human
ftomach cannot accommodate itfelf to ardent
fpirit, and dyfpeptic fymptoms are the early
figns of its being hurtful. The nervous, vil-
lous, and mufcular coats, the gaftric and mucous follicles of the ftomach, inftead of feeling
it neceffary for their functions, by every repetition of the draught, refift it the more
till at laft digeftion is overcome, a fixed
difeafe takes place in thefe organs, and the
fibres become hard and infenfible. It is true,
that during all thefe corporeal ailments the
mind is gradually forming a bad habit; it receives pleafure from the firft, but the body
nothing but difeafe and pain. We daily fee
in all parts of the world, men, who by pro-
fligacy and hard drinking, have brought
themfelves to a jail; yet if we confult the regifter of the prifon, it does not appear that
any of thefe habitual drunkards die by being
forced to lead fober lives. If at any time an
inebriate dies after he has been compelled to
temperance, his death is not to be attributed
to the want of fpirituous potation, but to the
too long continuance of it, which rendered
his difeafe incurable. The whole of thefe
arguments

arguments tend to prove that vinous ſtimulus
may be ſafely relinquiſhed *at once ;* the debility
of the body, if any exiſts, is then to be cured
by whatever may reſtore the weakened organs.
In moſt caſes nature will effect this, as theſe
organs have only been exhauſted by unnatural means.

But, in attempting to ſubtract the vinous
potation by little and little, a difficulty ariſes
which every one converſant with the ſubject
muſt have obſerved.   As ſoon as the limited
portion of liquor is ſwallowed, an agreeable
glow is experienced ; and by it ſo grateful
a feeling is conveyed to the mind, which in
an inſtant connects the chain of habit, that is
our duty to break.   This glow and feeling
are aſſociated in the patient's mind with all
thoſe pleaſurable ſenſations he has been accuſtomed to receive from his former bumper.
He therefore reaſons with himſelf that he
finds much relief ; and as he is aware that
the effect of the preſent doſe will only be of
ſhort duration, he muſt take another to pro-
long his reverie, and ward off ſome intruding
care.   With a ſecond glaſs he finds more
pleaſing objects preſented to his imagination,

N   and

and then he is urged to try a third. His de-
preſſed ſpirits, fears, and apprehenſions have
now vaniſhed : he is ſo happy within himſelf
that he deſpiſes fortune, and views the world
with contempt ; thus he goes on, libation
after libation, till he ſinks into a drunken
ſlumber.

> The happieſt he of all that e'er were mad,
> Or are or ſhall be, could this folly laſt.

The morning viſit of his phyſician will be
introduced with the inquiry about the quantity of wine drank yeſterday, and how he
ſlept in the night ? He will probably tell his
phyſician very frankly, that he rather exceeded his allowance, but ſlept well. But the
morning account ; ate no breakfaſt, pain
about the region of the liver worſe, great
flatulence, cardialgia, thirſt, headach, &c.
Such is the tenor of theſe conſultations, repeated day after day ; the patient muſt be
treated *ſecundum artem*, and nature is drove
out of the houſe. Dr. Lettſom, in his little
work on Drunkenneſs, tells us of a man that
dropped a bit of ſealing-wax into his dram-
glaſs every time he drank, till he filled it, and
by this means gradually got the better of his
habit.

habit. Whatever truth may be in this narrative, furely neither Dr. Lettfom or any other phyfician could be childifh enough to imitate it; for there could be no danger in filling the glafs at once, if the cure of the patient depended on that.

Again, are not habits of drunkennefs more often produced by mental affections than corporeal difeafes? I apprehend few people will doubt the truth of this. Does not the inebriate return to his potation rather to raife his fpirits, and exhilarate the mind, than to fupport and ftrengthen the body? The difeafes of the body, if unattended with dejecjection, have no need of vinous ftimulus; and three-fourths of the human race recover daily from all the ftages of debility without ever having recourfe to it. With drunkards therefore my opinion is, and confirmed by much experience, that wine, malt liquor, and fpirits, in every form, ought *at once* to be taken from them.

I have mentioned above the neceffity of ftudying the patient's temper and character, that we may acquire his confidence. Thefe will lead us to the particular caufe, time, and

place

place of his love of the bottle. The danger
of continuing his career may be then calmly
argued with him, and fomething propofed
that will effectually wean his affections from
it, and ftrenuoufly engage his attention. This
may be varied according to circumftances, and
muft be left to the difcretion of the phyfician.
" Mutatio loci, fi ex doloribus cordis, vel ad-
" verfis fortunæ aut amoris malum increvit,
" plurimum proderit. Hunc caftra et arma;
" hunc mufæ omnes; hunc artes elegantes;
" hunc rus amænum; illum venatio et variæ
" exercitationes fuaviter occupabunt; hunc
" negotia magis feria non male detinebunt.
" Et breviter cupiditas vini iifdem modis vin-
" cenda, diftantia et abfentia, quibus amator
" immitem dominam e pectore fuo pellit *."

In order to ftrengthen the body if debilitated, general remedies, as commonly employed, may be reforted to; fuch as the cold
bath, chalybeate waters, exercife in the open
air, condiments, vigorous diet, &c.

The waters of Bath are in confiderable re-
pute for their efficacy in recruiting the worn-
down conftitution of inebriates. But this

* Differtatio de Ebrietate, &c. p. 38. Edin. 1788.

means of relief can only be obtained by the
wealthy : the greater part of our patients
muft be content with cheaper remedies at
home. To thofe who can afford a journey
to Bath, for the purpofe of ufing its waters, I
can have no objection to the trial. Thefe
waters are now found, by the fuperior chemical analyfis of Dr. Gibbes, to contain iron
in a very diffufed ftate ; from which it is fair
to fuppofe their medical qualities chiefly arife.
This city alfo affords many elegant amufements, that may be confoling to a man who
has juft forfaken an unkind attachment.
That fpecies of *etiquette* which one is forced
to go through in fafhionable circles, and
among trifling entertainments, may, on particular people, have a powerful influence in
introducing new trains of thinking. The
hours are there well adapted to the comfort
of invalids. I would recommend people
who vifit this gay watering-place to keep a
diary of their pleafures and acquaintance.
They will find there a great variety of medical characters, probably the whole that are
mentioned in the *Iatrologia* of Dr. Beddoes.
But it is to be remembered that all this regi-

N 3   men

men will be in vain without a firm refolution
to perfevere in the chafteft temperance. It is
furprifing what nature will effect in the cure
of thofe violent dyfpeptic and hepatic affections which have been induced by intoxication, when the inordinate ufe of wine has
ceafed. Nay, thofe difeafes, when pronounced incurable, have fometimes yielded in a
few months to a plain diet and water beverage: Nothing, therefore, can be more en-
couraging to perfons who refolve firmly to
lead a regular and fober life.

The chief complaints which require medicine are of the dyfpeptic kind. The pain
and uneafinefs which they create is almoft
conftant ; and if accompanied with a hypochondriacal difpofition, nothing can be more
haraffing. It is always neceffary in fuch cafes
to correct the acidity prevailing in the ftomach and bowels ; which may be done by
Pulv. chel. comp. Pulv. cretæ comp. Mag.
uft. Aq. calcis, &c. Acidity with flatulence
often produces fpafmodic pains and twitches,
as they are called, as well as that irregular
and tumultuous motion of the inteftines called
borborrygmi. Bitters are readily combined
with

with thefe anti-acids, fuch as colombo, quaf-
fia, chamœmelum, &c.; they likewife im-
pede fermentation in the ftomach, and alfo
correct acidity. Iron, in its moft fuitable
ftate, for the form ought to be ftudied, given
in fmall quantity, and continued long, is
juftly celebrated in thefe cafes. I would have
the belly preferved in a foluble condition by
gentle laxatives; but all the harfher purga-
tives muft be avoided: if the diet can be fo
conducted as to fuperfede the ufe of medicine
in regulating this difcharge, fo much the
better. The cramps and fpafms which fo
often attend the weakened ftomach are readily relieved by æther. vitr. and opium, with
other ftimulants; but thefe generally yield
when the acidity is overcome. The phyfician, in directing his *formula*, will cautioufly
avoid every preparation that has ardent fpirit
in its compofition. I have feen and known
many inftances where the moft naufeous and
fetid tinctures were devoured with an avidity
not to be conceived, when it was found
that they were compounded of brandy. The
tafte of the mouth on fuch occafions has little
to do in exciting the defires of the patient:

there

there is a *vacuum* in fenfation, if I may fo
term it, that can be fupplied with nothing
but the vinous ftimulus while the habit remains, and the mind not earneftly in purfuit of fomething that can engage it.

The dyfpnœa, or fhortnefs of breath of
drunkards, is of two kinds. The one is fym-
pathetic with affections of the ftomach, liver,
heart, &c.; the other ufually precedes and
attends hydrothorax, and a general difpofition
to dropfy. It is a moft diftreffing fymptom,
as the maladies which it accompanies are
feldom curable; opiates, and æther. vit. give
temporary eafe. Some years ago I attended
an old gentleman of feventy-two, who laboured under a fevere dyfpnœa and general
dropfy. They were induced by *tippling* gin
and water, a phrafe very well applied to that
frequent recourfe to fpirit and water which
fome people practife without getting drunk.
This gentleman had a remarkable recovery,
from the exhibition of fquills, prepared as directed in the 3d vol. of *Medicina Nautica*,
article Phthifis. In the fpace of a year he
had a relapfe, and was cured in the fame
manner, but he never gave up his grog.
He lived to eighty-four.

In

In thofe vifceral obftructions, fuch as the tubercular or fchirrous liver, I am averfe to all fevere mercurial courfes. Indeed mercury in any form has feldom appeared to me to be of any fervice beyond its action in keeping the bowels open, where coftivenefs was to be guarded againft. I conceive the frame of an habitual drunkard to have been fo much exhaufted by inordinate and unnatural ftimuli, that it has long been my practice to commit him to the regimen of children, fuch as a diet of milk, and other kinds of nourifhment of the mildeft quality. In fhort, inftead of withdrawing the bottle by thofe flow degrees which have been long recommended by phyficians, my plan of *cure* is at once to take from him every thing that is highly ftimulating; to put him on food in direct oppofition to his former modes of living, and confign him to the lap of nature as if his exiftence were to pafs through a fecond infancy. Indeed the reformed drunkard muft be confidered as a regenerated being.

I have attended two cafes of difeafed liver within thefe few months from frequent fpirituous potation, although neither of them were
deemed

deemed intemperate drinkers. They both proved fatal, and were in the last stage of debility before I was consulted. One of them more liable to dyspepsia, laboured under jaundice, and the hue of the skin before death, as well as the urine, was nearly black. The other suffered from hydrothorax, though both had dropsy. Inebriates who have been corpulent, I think are more than others, liable to *hydrops pectoris*. Obesity by extending the cellular substance, when the adipose cells have been membrane, may pave the way to a greater halation and diminished absorption at the same time.

In the cases just mentioned the disease of the liver had been very slow in its progress, and without giving much pain. Indeed this viscus, notwithstanding its important office in digestion and sanguification, appears to be endued with little sensibility. When calculi are lodged in the ducts, acute pain is sometimes felt, but all its other diseases create little uneasiness. In icterus when the bile is carried in considerable quantity into the circulation, there is an unusual torpor of feeling and sluggishness of motion throughout the body.

body. Can the bile affect the oxygenation of the blood when abforbed in this manner? Might not this diminished fenfibility be owing to the abftraction of oxygene? Are hepatic obftructions induced by vinous potation, fimilar in appearance to thofe produced by hepatitis in tropical climates? Mercury fo fuccefsfully exhibited by Bontius, and others fince his time, in the difeafe of the Eaft Indies, has not, to my knowledge, ever relieved the tubercular affection from hard drinking.

The conftipation of bowels which follows intoxication, for a fingle paroxyfm may be owing to increafed abforption from vinous ftimulus; and diarrhœa may be caufed by the inverted motion of the lacteals, by the increafed action of exhalants and mucous glands, and alfo by the increafed periftaltic motion of the inteftines that hurries on their contents. The conftipation which attends habitual ebriety may arife from a weaker periftaltic motion, or deficiency of bile; the diarrhœa from diminished abforption, by the lacteals becoming torpid; the cure therefore can only be effected by removing the primary caufe of the mifchief.

Having

Having always directed my curative indications of habitual temulency chiefly to the state of the patient's mind, much may be frequently done by rousing particular passions, such as a parent's love for his children, the jealousy attached to character, the desire of fame, the pride of reputation, family pride, &c. I have seen a lovely infant force tears from a drunken father, when nothing else could affect him, though he was afterwards reclaimed. The good sense and management of an amiable wife, we know, will often accomplish wonders. The practice I would wish to inculcate, in taking advantage of the patient's temper and feelings, is nicely illustrated by the following fact: A friend of mine an eminent physician, in the north, was consulted by a gentleman on the subject of correcting an unfortunate attachment to the bottle, in the wife of his bosom. They formally sat down to deliberate, and the doctor listened with much patience to all the ways and means that had been devised by the distressed and affectionate husband to reclaim his *cara sposa*. So much had been done, and so many expedients tried in vain, that the physician declared, nothing further could be attempted,

attempted, but to place a hogſhead of brandy before her, and let her drink till *ſhe gave up the ghoſt!* The laſt part of the ſentence was pronounced with conſiderable emphaſis. It ſo happened that the lady ſuſpecting the ſubject of conſultation to be herſelf, was concealed in an adjoining room, and overheard every word. The words of the phyſician ſtrongly affected her; her pride was wounded, and her reſentment rouſed to the higheſt pitch imaginable. In the whirlwind of paſſion the chain of habit was broke in an inſtant; female delicacy reſumed its aſcendancy over her actions; and from that moment ſhe abjured the intoxicating charm. I am ſorry to add my honeſt friend was never after beheld with complaiſance by the fair convert, though he had proved to be her beſt benefactor.

In May laſt I was requeſted to viſit a reſpectable tradeſman, whom I found labouring under ſevere dyſpeptic complaints, depreſſion of ſpirits, great apprehenſion, and, at times, alienation of mind. For my two or three firſt viſits I was unable to divine the cauſe of ſuch extraordinary ſymptoms. But in the
course

courfe of attendance it at laft came out that
he had lately been much addicted to the
bottle. I could now take my ground to advantage; and in a long converfation with
him, he told me that fomething lay heavy on
his mind. He then related what it was: he
had fome months before been in a company
where one of his particular friends, in an un-
becoming manner, traduced the character of
another, and which ftrongly affected him.
This circumftance preyed upon his memory;
he could neither fleep or reft for it; and he
had recourfe to drinking to quiet the tumult
of his fpirits, and agitation of mind. Being
now informed of all the particulars of this
curious hallucination, with much difficulty I
at laft perfuaded him to relinquifh his liquor.
He kept his refolution for fome days, when
he relapfed, drank a confiderable quantity,
and next morning early all his horrors returned. About nine o'clock I found him
quite frantic; and he even fpoke of deftroying himfelf. He had now all the fymptoms of
phrenitic delirium, or *brain fever*. Being a
ftrong hale man I ordered venæfection; and
blood to the amount of twenty-four ounces was
taken

taken from him. He became quiet immediately; slept sound the succeeding night, and
only complained of weakness in the morning.
I now reasoned with him at my visits instead
of plying him with medicine: he listened
to my admonitions with great attention;
thanked me, even to tears, for the signal
change which my arguments had made upon
him, and happily regained his usual serenity
of mind.—I was much pleased with the successful issue of this case; for at first none
ever appeared more likely to terminate in
permanent madness.

Having now finished my method of treating and correcting the habit of intoxication,
as far as my own experience has warranted
me, I shall deliver my sentiments on what
appears to me the best method of *treating the
drunken Paroxysm.*

As the Materia Medica does not supply
any thing as yet known for correcting the
inebriating power of alkohol, the *cure of the
paroxysm* will turn very much in evacuating
it from the stomach; which must be best
done by throwing in quantities of lukewarm
water, and provoking vomiting. Acids, it is

7   true,

true, have been faid to prove very efficacious
in deftroying the ftimulant power of ardent
fpirit by chemical union, thereby altering its
nature. It has been a common practice to
exhibit acids to obviate the effect of large
dofes of opium: but it is doubtful whether
ever much good was done by their affiftance.
If this is at all a chemical queftion, it will not
be eafy to explain the mode of action of thefe
fubftances with opium. I would therefore,
at all times, prefer the method of dilution,
and provoking vomiting, if poffible. It is remarked in a former part of this effay that
death is fometimes fo fudden after the deglu-
tition of a large quantity of raw or undiluted
fpirit, that no time is given to call in medical
affiftance. Neverthelefs this practice is fo
fimple as to be eafily carried into effect by
any perfon prefent: but I am ignorant whether any rules on the fubject have been publifhed by the Humane Society.

Should the drunken man have fo far loft
the power of fenfe and motion as to be unable to help himfelf, he ought to be placed
either in an armed chair, where he cannot
fall, or laid in a bed with the head erect,
inclining

inclining a little to the one fide, for the purpofe of facilitating vomiting. The neckcloth
ought to be taken off, and the collar of the
fhirt unbuttoned. The doors and windows
of the room ought to be thrown open, for a
free ventilation; all vifitors beyond affiftants
muft be excluded, and whatever may add to the
heat of the body is to be carefully avoided.

If his face is much fwoln, and unufually
fluſhed or bloated; if his breathing is fterte-
rous, with the eyes fixed and veffels turgid,
there is danger of an inftant fit of apoplexy.
How far bleeding with the lancet, cupping
the temples, or applying leeches, for the
purpofe of relieving the brain, are to be
depended upon, I cannot well determine.
I have tried bleeding, and the patient has
recovered that fit; but in a few hours
another one has carried him off. If, however, thefe means fhould be attempted, attention muft be paid to the ftrength and age of
the patient, and to the degree of comatofe
fymptoms, fo as to regulate the quantity of
blood neceffary to be taken away. Which
being done the ftomach is to be quickly un-
loaded; and as the delay in exhibiting eme-

o   tics

tics might be fatal, the beſt means of accom-
pliſhing this is by introducing a feather or
any ſuitable ſubſtance into the mouth, and
tickling the fauces, till the contents of that
viſcus are all evacuated*.

I am well aware that there are phyſicians
who may heſitate to direct vomiting in the
manner which I have propoſed. Vomiting,
under an impending apoplexy, has been conſidered a dangerous practice ; as during the
inverted action of the ſtomach, and the col-
lapſed ſtate of lungs, by a long inſpiration,
the blood is accumulated in the blood-veſſels
of the brain, and thus a greater hazard of
their diſtenſion, rupture and effuſion from
them take place. That ſuch things might
happen during the effort of vomiting I do
not mean to diſpute : but I have long made
the obſervation that ſpontaneous vomiting is
a certain relief when there is every ſign of
inſtant apoplexy. I therefore conceive it fair

* Si ebrius quiſpiam repente aphonius fiat, convulſus
moritur, niſi febre corripiatur, aut ubi, ad horam perve-
nerit, qua crapulæ ſolvuntur vocem recuperit.

Hip. Aphor. v. ſect. 5.

Qui ebrius obmutuit, is fere nervorum diſtentione con-
ſumitur, niſi aut febris acceſſit, aut eo tempore, quo ebrie-
tas ſolvi debet, loqui cœpit. Cel. De Med. l. ii. c. 6.

to

to imitate that effort by art. Indeed those gentlemen who have cavilled most at this practice have produced no fact to controvert it : their dislike to it rests solely on theoretical opinions. To these opinions, fortunately, the operations of nature are not obliged to bend : for if we are to suppose it dangerous to evacuate the loaded stomach of the inebriate, vomiting, at any time, must be considered as an operation not only inexpedient but to a certainty hurtful.

The means of exciting vomiting, I have said above, are so simple, that any person might accomplish it, as in the following instance : A gentleman returning home on a dark night stumbled over something soft in the street, which induced him to examine what it was, when it proved to be a man most insensibly drunk. Not wishing to leave him to the hazard of being trod upon by a horse or carriage, he waited for the next passenger, who kindly took him on his back. They carried him to the first light which they saw, which proved to be his own house, and where his mother was anxiously waiting his return from a corporation feast. The man

was

was to all appearance dying: but one of the gentlemen having perufed my thefis, thought, if any thing could fave him, it was by unloading the ftomach, which was effected by forcing down warm water. This timely expedient brought him quickly to his fenfes, and he was fnatched from the jaws of death. I firmly believe that many human beings might be faved were equal humanity exercifed for the recovery of drunkards in fimilar conditions.

I would alfo recommend the bowels to be immediately emptied by glyfters. Common falt, to the amount of two table-fpoonfuls, diffolved in a pint of water, bloodwarm, can be eafily procured, and will act quickly.

Throughout the whole paroxyfm the application of cold water, rectified fpirit of wine, or æther, to the head and temples, is proper. Although it may be difficult to explain the *modus operandi* of thefe articles, I am well convinced of their utility; but the cold produced by their evaporation from the head, may in a great meafure account for their good effects. The affufion of cold water, or

the

the shower-bath, when it can be procured, might be still more beneficial.

" Senatorem Britannicum celeberrimum, " (non magis spectabilem elegantia orationis, " quam frequentia ebrietatis,) fertur, gravem " vino, mantile aqua frigida bene madefac- " tum circum caput conftringere, in lectulum " se recipere; et mane expergefactum ad " curiam pergere, mirabile dictu! sine capitis " dolore, vel languore, vel laffitudine aut " animi aut corporis, ad dicendum semper " paratum*."

Analagous to the use of the wet kerchief bound about the head, is the *clay cap*, some- times tried in maniacal cases. Whatever moderates the heat and velocity of the cir- culation in the brain, would seem to be beneficial in both diseases.

Sudden immersion of the body in cold water has often brought a drunkard to his senses. I have frequently known this happen in His Majesty's ships, where seamen, in a state of stupid intoxication, have fallen over- board; they are generally sober when picked up. The case of the miller mentioned in

* Differt. De Ebrietate, p. 41.

a former

a former part of this Effay, fupports the opinion. Buffon fays, " Among the favages " in the Ifthmus of America, the women " throw their drunk hufbands into the rivers, " in order the more fpeedily to remove the " effects of intoxication *." This practice among thefe favages was probably tried at firft as a punifhment, but having obferved its good effects it was continued as a remedy. The cuftom of *ducking* a drunken hufband, common enough in different parts of this ifland, had moft likely a fimilar origin. It is much to be lamented that our fair country-women do not exercife their privilege much oftener. But it is to be remembered, that there are limits to the practice of cold im-merfion, whether local or general. The pa-roxyfm of ebriety is to be diftinguifhed by two ftages, each exhibiting very different fymptoms. The firft ftage comprehends that train of fymptoms which fubfifts during the ftimulant power of the wine, fuch as heat of body, full pulfe, flufhed countenance, &c. The fecond ftage includes thofe figns of de-bility which fucceed; the body is cold, the

* Chap. on Infancy, vol, ii.

pulfe

pulfe weak, and the countenance pale. To the firſt ſtage, the cool regimen and eva- cuating plan are chiefly to be confined; nay, it is likely theſe would do much harm when the debility commences, for expoſure to cold, and ſleeping on damp ground after in- toxication, have brought on many mortal diſeaſes. It is under theſe circumſtances, I think, that the inflammatory affections are produced; the body being firſt weakened and chilled, and then improperly brought near great fires, or into warm rooms, is all at once plied with every thing heating.

An officer of my own acquaintance having often heard that cooling the head would re- lieve ebriety, when in the ſecond ſtage of the paroxyſm, plunged his head into a bucket of cold water, as being the moſt effectual way, was ſoon after ſeized with phrenitis, or *brain fever* as vulgarly called, of which he died in a few days. Cold water applied to the head is not therefore a ſafe remedy at all times for the head-ache of drunkards.

Perſons addicted to ebriety are often found in the ſtreets and highways, and ſometimes in theſe ſituations expoſed to the moſt inclement weather.

weather. Were they to remain long in that condition in severe frosts they must run great hazard of perishing; for as soon as the second stage of the paroxysm commences, the body becomes feeble, the circulation of the blood languid, and the vital powers so exhausted that no great time would be required for the complete extinction of the living principle. It is to be suspected that most of the travellers who perish among snow, are of this description; fool-hardy, under the false courage of dram-drinking, they sally out in the dark to explore their way, and quickly lose the road, from the change of objects, which falling snow, or snow already fallen, occasions. The dram in this situation of distress only helps to accelerate death, it assists in bringing on drowsiness and sleep, which leaves the body to be sooner weakened by the cold, and the benighted traveller never wakes again!

If, however, signs of life appear when the person is found, great caution is necessary; lest, by attempting to recover him by strong spirits, and carrying him too near a fire, you extinguish the small remains of the vital principle.

ciple. Here all the means and the pre-
cautions ufually taken for the recovery of
froft-bitten limbs will be neceffary. The
hands, arms, feet, and legs, may at firft be
rubbed with fnow, or wafhed with cold water,
then wiped dry, and the patient put to bed.
The firft thing to be given by the mouth,
may be a little warm milk, and as the heat of
the body increafes, fomething more ftimulant
may be added. The great object to be attended to, is to cherifh the flender remains
of life by the gentleft ftimuli, for the ftronger
would tend to deftroy them. The future
ftrength of the body is to be recruited by
meafures fuited to the condition of the fyftem, which need not be detailed here.

It might perhaps be confidered by fome as
too great a compliment to inftruct the drunkard how to correct morning head-ache and
fick ftomach. I have quoted before the lines
of Horace which apply to this fubject.
Something relifhing is ufually ferved up on
this occafion, fuch as falted fifh, ham, falted,
or fmoke-dried meat, &c. Kitchen falt is a
very grateful ftimulus to a ftomach weakened
by excefs. Dr. Cullen, in his Lectures

on Dyspepsia, used to say, that he had found it prove anti emetic when every thing else failed.

> " Si nocturna tibi noceat potatio vini,
> " Ex eodem mane bibas, medicina fuerit."
>
> SANCTOR.

Acidity, gastrodynia, &c. are to be relieved by anti-acids and stimulants. Dr. Home says, " Calor lecti, equitatio et elixir vitrioli, " nauseam hesterni Bacchi abigunt *." There are, perhaps, some who will prefer a morning ride, or other kinds of exercise in the open air, or the cold bath, to all kinds of medicine.

I have certainly known and heard of instances of ebriety being quickly changed into sobriety by fear, danger, excessive joy or grief, acute pain, and probably by whatever means sudden impressions are made on our sentient system. But as these means cannot easily be imitated by our art. it would tend to no useful purpose to offer any speculations on the mode of action.

As a fit of ebriety leaves the body dull, languid, weak, and prone to numerous dif-

* Principia Medicinæ.

eases,

eafes, great caution ought to be taken in ex-
pofing it in that ftate to marfh effluvium, to
humidity, cold, or any kind of contagion,
whether of fever or others.

———————

I fhall now conclude this Effay with the
following admonition : Let all thofe perfons,
whofe conftitutions have any predifpofition to
the difeafes mentioned in the catalogue, beware how they get drunk, or fall into the
habit of intoxication. For this predifpofition
will haften the approach of that difeafe, that
muft in the end terminate their exiftence.
Such perfons as Celfus finely advifes, " Suf-
" pecta habere fua bona debere."

———Not poppy nor mandragora,
Nor all the drowfy fyrups of the world,
Shall ever med'cine thee to that fweet fleep
Which thou ow'dft yefterday.   SHAKESPEAR.

THE END.

BOOKS *lately published by the same Author.*

1. Medicina Nautica: An Essay on the Diseases of Seamen, comprehending the History of Health in the Fleet from 1793 to 1802. 3 vols. 1 l. 3 s.

2. Observations on Scurvy. 2d Edition, 4 s.

3. Medical and Chemical Essays. 2d Edition, 3 s. 6d.

4. Suspiria Oceani: A Monody on the Death of Admiral Earl Howe, K. G. 2 s.

Printed by A. Strahan,
Printers-Street.